Breath for the Soul

"Combining modern science and ancient wisdom, *Breath for the Soul* offers evidence-based approaches to practicing self-care. Whether you need to heal or to stay well, this book offers practical advice, encouraging reminders, and inspiring thoughts that speak to your physical and spiritual nature. In *Breath for the Soul*, Patterson and Nichols offer ways that provide structure, flexibility, and inspiration for you as you practice self-care that becomes a lifestyle, not a checklist of things to do."

Harold G. Koenig, M.D.
Professor of Psychiatry & Behavioral Sciences
Director, Center for Spirituality, Theology and Health
Duke University Medical Center, Durham, North Carolina
Author of *Handbook of Religion and Health*

"*Breath for the Soul* offers is a decidedly unique guide for individuals who wish to experience greater wellness. With her medical background and expertise in integrative medicine, Dr. Patterson offers explanations for simple yet effective self-care practices. Phyllis follows these explanations with Christian-based spiritual insights. Their voices interweave to create a gentle fabric of self-care which will provide comfort and calm."

Lise Alschuler, ND
Professor of Clinical Medicine
University of Arizona –
Andrew Weil Center for Integrative Medicine
Author of *The Definitive Guide to Thriving After Cancer*

"Authors Jan Patterson and Phyllis Nichols introduce us to *Breath for the Soul*, in which they emphasize the importance of finding oneself. They remind us of our responsibility to promote self-care, and provide guidance on achieving personal goals of balance and well-being. The strategies outlined by Patterson and Nichols are easy and practical approaches intent on equipping us with techniques to strengthen our resiliency to life's challenges and stressors. *Breath for the Soul* seamlessly describes how to enhance and improve our four pillars of self-care: breath, movement, nutrition, and spirit. The valuable guidance offered through-out each chapter is actionable, sustainable, and can easily be incorporated into our daily lives. This book is an invaluable guide and practical approach to living in a world that continues to demand more of us while leaving little breathing room for us. This book serves as a valuable guide and practical approach to handle an inevitable part of life."

Charles C. Reed PhD, RN
VP/ACNO Center for Clinical Excellence
University Health

"For almost three decades I served as a Navy chaplain. It was common practice to transfer from ship to ship or unit to unit by helicopter. The flights were known as the 'holy helo.' For weeks, in one large, arduous, and dangerous operation for all involved, the flight designation changed. A physician and I joined together in the flights and the care for our troops. We were a two-person team subsequently dubbed 'body and soul.' It was appropriate. People are more than the sum of their 'parts.' The physical, psychological, and the spiritual dimensions of every person are complex and integrated. To live fully and as we were created, the whole person—'body and soul' or 'body and spirit'—must breathe or perish. Drawing on decades of professional and personal experiences that have survived the trials, traumas, and tragedies of life, the authors present compelling research and compassionate reflection that provide fresh breath and a second wind for weary souls. Read, breathe, and reflect with these perceptive authors—it will give you fresh air for your spirit."

Timothy J. Demy, Th.D., Ph.D.
Professor, U.S. Naval War College
Chaplain, U.S. Navy (Ret.)
Author of *Silent Nights, Silent Guns*

"This book is an evidence-based healer's manual that is also filled with spiritual wisdom. As an infectious disease doctor battling a pandemic, I have regularly benefitted from this type of body and soul-restoring breathing, meditation, good nutrition, use of essential oils, forest bathing and vigorous exercise. I especially welcome the voices of Phyllis and Jan as guides on the path to a healthy spirit—they bring healing to healers with courage and conviction."

Ruth Berggren MD, MACP, Infectious Disease Specialist
Professor of Medicine at Dartmouth Health and Geisel
School of Medicine
Director, Center for Medical Humanities & Ethics at the
University of Texas Health, San Antonio, TX

"The eye-opening, yet simple instructions and practical tools I learned from *Breath for the Soul* helped me rise above the pain, fatigue, and depression from the debilitating effects of my cancer treatments. It's no exaggeration to say this book was life changing for me."

George, CEO of a media corporation and cancer survivor

"This book honors all aspects of healing coming from our Great Physician and Creator!"

Nooshig Luz Salvador MD, MSOM, ABOIM, NCCAOM
Integrative Medicine and Palliative Medicine Physician,
Herbalist and Acupuncturist, Ethicist

"Congratulations on your important insights and contributions, which are fundamental and empowering."

Larry Dossey, MD
New York Times best-selling author of *Healing Words*

Breath for the Soul is a beautifully written book blending integrative medicine with spirituality. The authors provide practical guidance on how to improve one's mental and physical wellbeing in daily life or while confronting personal challenges using breathing techniques, movement, nutrition and acknowledging one's spirituality. As a Transplant Surgeon, I face many daily stressors including the emotional extremes faced by my patients as they navigate their disease and their unpredictable wait for a lifesaving organ transplant. I am a better and healthier person after reading *Breath for the Soul*, and I will recommend this book to my patients and friends as they face their own challenges as the lessons learned will help bring presence and beauty to their lives even during despair. I truly believe these lessons will help one live a better life and heal a person no matter what the affliction might be."

Francisco G. Cigarroa, MD
Director of Transplantation
Carlos and Malu' Alvarez University
Distinguished Chair in Transplantation
UT Health San Antonio, TX

Breath for the Soul

Self-Care As a Way to Wellness

Dr. Jan Evans Patterson
and
Phyllis Clark Nichols

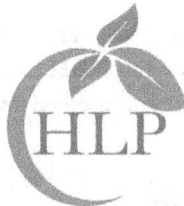

HLP

Healing Leaves Publishing

Published by Healing Leaves Publishing

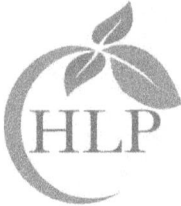

Healing Leaves Publishing

ISBN: 979-8-9869877-0-5 (paperback)
ISBN: 979-8-9869877-1-2 (ebook)

Authors' Note

This book is intended to provide useful information on the topics discussed. It is not intended to diagnose or treat any medical condition. Please be sure to discuss decisions regarding your health—including breathing exercises, nutrition, and movement—with your own health-care professional.

For Tom, Evan, Ivy, and Will,
with thanks for love and inspiration.

and

For Bill, whose strength and resilience
inspire me every day.

Contents

Introduction

We live in an incredible time in human history. But even with all the advances in medicine, science, and technology, we humans are still dealing with some age-old problems—those of stress, anxiety, depression, and grief. *Breath for the Soul* addresses these issues and will provide you with steps for self-care—things you can do for yourself to help alleviate the symptoms and put you on the path to wellness.

You might be asking this question: how is it that a medical doctor and professor recognized in infectious diseases and a seminary-trained inspirational writer and novelist collaborated to write this book? The answer is that we have been good friends for over twenty-five years, we have dealt personally with the issues we address in this book, and we desire to help others with what we have learned from our perspectives and knowledge bases.

From Dr. Jan

I had been practicing medicine for about thirty years when I experienced a series of personal losses that I will elaborate on within this book. As I have already explained to many patients, I noted for myself that while conventional medicine can do many great things, it is challenging to treat stress, anxiety, depression, and grief with this approach alone. With conventional medicine, most health-care professionals are trained to offer a pill. This approach is often needed; it can improve health and be lifesaving. Yet, including the treatment of the whole person—what Phyllis and I refer to as the *soul* that includes mind and spirit as well as the body—is often overlooked. None of these self-care measures we discuss are intended to take the place of medication that your doctor prescribes. They are intended to be integrated with traditional medicine that you may need as determined by your doctor.

As Rachel Naomi Remen, MD, said, "It is not that we have a soul but that we are a soul." Many times, the difficulties of life can distance us from our soul, from our true selves. There are ways that we can reawaken the sense of our soul. These are among the self-care strategies that we will discuss.

My journey into complementary therapies began when I was introduced to essential oils by my massage therapist. I found that I benefitted from essential-oil support for mood and emotions as well as a number of other complaints including allergies, insomnia, indigestion, and more. (Essential oils are not FDA-approved to treat, prevent, diagnose, or cure any diseases.) Having a scientific background, I wanted to understand more about how essential oils worked, and so I studied texts and took many hours of instruction to become registered as an aromatherapist. As I experienced the benefits of essential oils for myself and others, it occurred to me that there must be other complementary therapies that could help me and other people.

I researched additional therapies and discovered the field of integrative medicine. The field was pioneered by Andrew Weil, MD, and is an approach to medicine that involves the whole person, including body, mind, and spirit—the soul. Integrative medicine is informed by evidence and is so named for the integration of complementary and holistic therapies with conventional ones. I completed a fellowship in integrative medicine at the Andrew Weil Center for Integrative Medicine at University of Arizona, where I learned about mind-body medicine, complementary and alternative practices, botanicals and dietary supplements, nutritional health, and integrative approaches to multiple medical conditions.

What I learned was helpful to me and others, and I began to apply integrative practices in my clinic, and also to work with our hospital system to establish an integrative medicine program. I began to see successes with this approach and the appreciation of patients and staff who were encouraged and supported by these modalities.

Much of the integrative approach involves self-care. And as I sought to instruct others in self-care practices, I began to think in terms of recurring themes of four pillars of self-care:

- Breath
- Movement

- Nutrition
- Spirit

All of these benefit from mindfulness—the practice of being present in the moment and undistracted by ruminations of what happened yesterday or worries about what will happen later today or tomorrow.

Self-care strategies like intentional breathing, movement, nutrition, and spiritual connection can be extremely powerful and beneficial. Intentional breathing is an effective way to invoke our relaxation response. Likewise, there is increasing evidence that movement is beneficial for our moods as well as our physical health.[1] In regard to nutrition, the Standard American Diet (SAD), high in inflammatory foods, processed foods, and sugar, is failing us. The Mediterranean Diet and the Anti-Inflammatory Diet offer lifestyles with healthier yet delicious foods that can make us feel better mentally, emotionally, and physically. And there is scientific evidence that people who embrace spirituality, as defined by a personal connection to a higher power, actually have a more activated brain—an awakened brain that offers more resilience and combats depression.[2] Quieting practices such as mindfulness and time in nature prepare us for spiritual awareness.

I wanted to partner with my longtime friend Phyllis Clark Nichols for this project to enrich the spiritual component. Phyllis is a gifted inspirational author and an expert musician. She is also one of the kindest, most insightful, and spiritually attuned people I know. She and her husband, Dr. Bill Nichols (a brilliant artist, author, and retired minister), have been spiritual mentors to me and my family for many years.

We will discuss evidence for each of the pillars of breath, movement, nutrition, and spirit, as self-care strategies for stress, anxiety, depression, and grief—conditions we all encounter at times in our lives. Phyllis will have a spiritual illustration and interpretation for all of these to enrich our spiritual awareness.

From Phyllis

As a former executive for a national cable television network featuring programming on health and disability, I developed a growing interest in wellness and self-care, and I had the opportunity to meet many influential people who shared my interest. During those thirteen years in the health television field, I witnessed firsthand some shifts in health and medicine.

I grew up in a small southern town at a time in our nation's history when most people's views of health, medicine, and wellness were limited. If I became sick, I went to the doctor for a prescription and went home to follow the doctor's orders without question and without any sense of giving self-care. I believed it was the doctor's responsibility to cure me, and the prescription was the magic potion to make me well again. My only role was to follow the doctor's orders.

There was little sense of personal responsibility in caring for myself or for working toward wellness. The only mention of wellness I recall was the old adage, "An apple a day will keep the doctor away." All I learned of good nutrition was the food chart from health class in elementary school—which now turns out wasn't necessarily so healthy. And we were not told how important exercise was to our general health. Exercise was generally undertaken by athletes or someone trying to lose weight.

This was what I knew and experienced in my early life, but there were four factors that greatly influenced the change in my mindset: (1) personal illness, (2) relationships with many medical professionals who had a much larger view of health and medicine, (3) the explosion into the age of information and personal access via the internet to quality health-care data never before available to me, and (4) my belief that we humans are so much more than flesh and that there must be ways we can better care for our total selves.

Although I'd had much exposure to what was going on in the medical field through my job, when my husband, Bill, was diagnosed with his first life-threatening cancer in 2012, my need to learn became very personal and serious. That cancer was treated successfully with surgery. Then again, in 2018, Bill was diagnosed with another unrelated but life-threatening cancer. He was given weeks of chemotherapy followed by extensive surgery. We were determined to keep our lives as normal as possible. Cancer did not change who we were, it just changed what we did for a time.

During those months after his second surgery, we were grateful for excellent medical care, and I began reading and researching to learn what we could do to participate in his ongoing care. Our goal was to get him healthy and for both of us to stay healthy. We had always been disciplined with our eating and exercise, but with gratitude for Dr. Jan, I was learning more about food as medicine and fuel, exercise as healing, the effective use of essential oils, and the importance of proper breathing. We experienced the value of mindfulness and the use of guided imagery during Bill's treatment and recovery.

At that same time, Dr. Jan was gaining knowledge and working toward establishing an integrative medicine practice. She introduced me to the use of essential oils, gave me books to read and study, and taught me how to make everything from aroma sticks to soothing balms and creams. I began to use them and see amazing results. My husband's digestive issues and allergies improved. I began to rid our house of anything toxic—cleaning supplies, garden chemicals, skin-care products, and shampoos that had harmful ingredients. Dr. Jan taught us breathing techniques and suggested other forms of exercise and the importance of movement even in the healing and recovery process after treatment and surgery.

I fear I flooded Dr. Jan's phone and email in-box at times with my excitement when we experienced good results from using these modalities. Since I wasn't a medical professional, I was somewhat reluctant to share my experiences with others. But I wanted to. I longed for my family and friends to step onto the path to wellness and to realize that these practices do work. I wanted them to enjoy the benefits of these modalities. I didn't want their children to grow up as I had, thinking that a prescription was magic and they had no responsibility in the care and health of their bodies. I wanted them to grow up to be healthier and to see that self-care is of great value.

Finally, within these pages, I have the opportunity to say these things and to share some of our experiences. That's the reason I am so excited about this project. *Breath for the Soul* is the book I wish I could have pulled from my bookshelf years ago. I had the great blessing of having Dr. Jan, who taught me so much about wellness and self-care at a time when I was in desperate need of that information. I had access to many books informing me about ways to give care to my body through diet and exercise. Our bookshelves were filled with devotional books, Bible commentaries, and self-help books in psychology that spoke to the needs of my spirit. But I found no one book that addressed the needs of my soul—the total person that I am. *Breath for the Soul* speaks to the needs of the total person—mind, body, and spirit, and it addresses specific ways that we can give care to our bodies and our spirits on our paths toward whole-ness and wellness.

From both of us

You will find *Breath for the Soul* rich in information and yet simple in giving very specific practices that work and that you can do at home for the most part without any substantial investment of money, only an investment of your time. These disciplines, if practiced consistently over time, will also improve your general well-being.

There is no one who has no need for self-care. Whether you're healthy and whole, receiving care, or giving care, you still need self-care. You do not have to be dealing with serious emotional issues or life-threatening disease to benefit from the practices you will learn in this book. Of course, we encourage you to consult with your own doctor as you make decisions that affect your health.

The book is organized into four parts addressing the topics of stress, anxiety, depression, and grief. Under each topic, we deal with the modalities of breath, movement, nutrition, and spirit. Dr. Jan opens each topic with the physiological explanation of how these issues affect your body and then gives detailed information about modalities you can use to ease your symptoms. Then Phyllis will add spiritual insights. You will hear from both of us in every chapter as we share personal experiences, tell stories of others, and explain how we use these modalities in our own self-care.

Breath for the Soul was a carefully chosen title. And in keeping with our purpose for the book, we have included a section we call *Inhale* at the end of each chapter. These are quotes, scriptures, and thoughts for you to ponder and breathe into your life. As with the physical breath, *Exhale* follows *Inhale* as we breathe out our prayers, our gratitude, and our requests for help and guidance as we take steps toward wellness. The last section in each chapter is a list of practical *Self-Care Steps* for action on your path to peace, calm, hope, and gratitude.

Finally, at the end of the book, we provide additional information, resources and references, recipes, and a way to develop your own self-care plan.

We believe humans are more than flesh. We believe that as God created humans and breathed into us His breath, He made us spiritual as well as physical beings. Matthew Lee Anderson, founder of Mere Orthodoxy, said, "You are a body. But you're a soul too. And your human flourishing is contingent upon being a soul-bodied thing."

God created us with certain needs or desires. Abraham Maslow, an American psychologist of the 1940s, has categorized these needs.[3] Our bodies have physical needs in order for them to exist on this planet: air, light, water, food, and rest. Humans also desire to feel safe and healthy, to feel cherished and respected, and to have purpose and a sense of their eternal security. For us to be whole, well, and healthy people physically and emotionally, these needs must be met, and God has provided ways to meet those needs.

Life and circumstances create situations where our needs are not met, and stress, anxiety, depression, and grief creep in. Sometimes they come crashing in, uninvited and unexpected. This book, unlike any other book we know, will provide the information that can help you to give self-care, easing your symptoms and restoring your feelings of wholeness and wellness.

No matter how we explain God's role in the way He created us, it all comes down to this: the eternal God gave us physical bodies and everything we need to take care of our bodies. But He also gave us the *more* in life—that which transcends and is above the physical. It is this *more* that gives our physical dimension meaning and value. And with His Spirit and our spirits, He has provided ways for us to experience the *more*.

We have firsthand knowledge of the benefit of spiritual experience in our lives. It has transformed difficulties and tragedies into hope and healing. It is affirming and not surprising to us to learn that there is even scientific evidence now of the tangible benefits of spirituality. Not only is a spiritual person more likely to find internal resources to counter the difficulties of life, structural and functional brain studies actually demonstrate a more awakened brain.[4] The spirituality that we share is based in the Judeo-Christian faith, and this is the perspective Phyllis will share with you in her reflections.

It is our hope that you will incorporate the aspects of intentional breathing, movement, nutrition, spirituality, and mindfulness that can work for you, and that you benefit from these steps to self-care in your journey through life. We pray that this book will encourage you to develop your own self-care plan on your way from stress to peace, from anxiety to calm, from depression to hope, and from grief to gratitude.

Jan E. Patterson, MD, MS, and Phyllis Clark Nichols

Part One

Self-Care for Stress

Step One

Let's Take a Breath

"The single most effective relaxation technique I
know is the conscious regulation of breath."

Dr. Andrew Weil

From Dr. Jan

It seems that stress is always there, surrounding us.
Waiting to engulf us. A stress response in the right
setting and right amount can be beneficial. It can help us
with physical and mental performance. Our ancestors
needed it when they were running from predators and
physically fighting for their lives.

When our body or mind detects a threat—physical or
emotional—our brain and autonomic (automatic)
nervous system respond and send messages to the
adrenal gland, which produces our body's cortisol
steroid and adrenaline. These substances increase
alertness, heart rate, and blood pressure and focus
attention on the perceived threat. At the same time,
functions such as digestion, sleep, growth, pleasure, and
development are put on hold until the perceived threat is
over.

So, while there is a time and place for the stress response to be helpful, chronic stress is bad for us. Decades ago, Hans Selye researched the effects of chronic stress.[1] He found that the body could adapt to ongoing stress with the physiological changes above—increased heart rate, blood pressure, and alertness—but eventually exhaustion and adverse effects occurred. While there have been many refinements in stress research since Selye's work, it's still true that continual stress is harmful—physically and mentally. It increases inflammation in our body and thus our risk for heart disease, diabetes, high blood pressure, indigestion, pain, anxiety, infertility, sleep disorders, and more. And it can cause us to overeat, plan poorly, and make bad decisions.

But it's hard to keep from being stressed. While we don't have to worry about predators chasing us like our ancestors did, our digital and fast-paced world surrounds us with stressors—deadlines at work, toxic people, traffic, fussy children, illness, financial worries, emails and texts that come throughout the day and evening... Where does it end?

Sometimes we are responsible for increasing the stressors ourselves. We learn to be productive in more and more ways and thus accomplish more tasks. As the adage goes, "If you want something done, ask a busy person." However, we can find ourselves spending time on tasks that are less important, even though we can do them efficiently, rather than time on tasks that really matter. We may put that work off but then never get it done. It can be helpful to decide what tasks really matter and release unimportant ones.

Our digital connections have multiplied some of these less important tasks and have made them pervasive throughout the day in our lives. With the continual connectedness through our smartphones, laptops, and computers, we are constantly looking at email, responding to texts, and checking social media. Cal Newport, an associate professor of computer science at Georgetown University, expounded on digital minimalism in his book *Digital Minimalism: Choosing a Focused Life in a Noisy World*.[2] This is a philosophy in which your online time is focused on activities that support the things you value and that omits those you do not. He suggests batching the check-ins with social media, based on your needs, to once daily or even once weekly. You can designate certain times of day to go through emails so that you are not continually checking them throughout the day.

Catherine Price's *How to Break Up with Your Phone* points out that social media and digital applications are designed to be addictive.[3] Constantly checking email and scrolling through social media can add to our stress, particularly with the vitriol that often circulates on social media. We have become accustomed to picking up our phones in a moment we don't have something else to do—even in the elevator or walking in the hall. Price discusses strategies to help us return to mindfulness, to take some deep breaths and just be present with where we are and what we are experiencing at the moment.

We think nothing of phone snubbing—phubbing—our family members and friends when we pull out our phones at meals and other times to distance ourselves from them. Price suggests strategies for "reclaiming our brain" and setting limits on our phone use with *phasts*, or designated phone-free times. These can be during our evening meal, when taking a walk outside, or during exercise time. Set your phone on airplane mode, Do Not Disturb, or even turn it off during these times. Price and others have also described a *digital sabbath* in which you take a full day away from your phone. She notes some helpful steps to prepare for this.

In any case, taking time to decrease our digital connections, increase mindfulness and focus on the present, engage in earnest conversations, and spend some time in solitude can help us destress.

Focusing our minds on our breath and using intentional breathing to breath more slowly, deeply, and regularly can help control our stress response.[4] This simple strategy tells our autonomic nervous system and brain, via the vagus nerve, that it is okay to turn off the stress response and turn on the relaxation response. The term *vagus* comes from the Latin word for wandering, and this nerve takes a wandering path from the brain to many organs in the body, including the lungs, heart, and gastrointestinal tract.

The tone of the vagus nerve can be measured by heart-rate variability. Take your pulse as you breathe in and out. You'll notice that your heart rate speeds up when you breathe in and slows down as you breathe out.

The greater the difference between your inhalation heart rate and your exhalation heart rate, the higher your heart-rate variability or your vagal tone. A higher vagal tone means a more responsive parasympathetic nervous system, or relaxation response. Another measure of vagal tone is your resting heart rate. In general, the higher the vagal tone, the lower your resting heart rate.

As we control our breathing intentionally by deep, slow, regular breathing, our bodies respond by slowing the heart rate and lowering the blood pressure. Our minds think more clearly, and we can make better decisions. We are more likely to be kind and less likely to be angry when dealing with people.

Intentional breathing can start simply with just following the breath. Notice your inhale and your exhale. Think about breathing slowly, deeply, through your nose if you can. Place one hand on your chest and one on your abdomen. Does your abdomen expand when you are breathing, or only your chest? We tend to use only chest breathing when we are stressed or upset. For your fullest breath and best relaxation response, include your abdomen in breathing. Make your exhale a little longer than your inhale. For instance, inhale for five counts and exhale for six counts.

Now, take a couple of breaths, and read on.

From Phyllis

Have you ever wanted to walk through the door after busy day, slam that door, and shut out the world and everyone and everything in it that has caused you stress? Oh, how we wish it worked that way. We cannot eliminate stress entirely from the dailyness of our days, and certainly not by just slamming a door. So, if we cannot eliminate or avoid the tension and pressure, we must learn to live with it.

When God made our bodies, He made them such that they need water, light, rest, food, and to breathe. He provided for those all needs. He knew there would be times when we'd require the chemicals that enable us to function better in times of stress. He also knew that we'd need relief from strain, and He gave us good minds, thoughts, practices, and natural resources to help us deal with stress.

If you look in the dictionary at the antonyms for the word *stress,* you'll find words like *peace, contentment,* and *serenity.* Sometimes, we think of peace and contentment as the absence of that thing that causes us such discontent. We think we'd have peace if we didn't have bills. If we didn't have such pressure at work. If we didn't have this unhealthy relationship that causes us so much pain. If we didn't have so much responsibility. If, if, if. Those *ifs* are not ever likely to be absent. The truth is this: the peace and contentment we long for are not the absence of anything.

Peace—real peace—is the presence of the One who made you and loves you. You are His fearfully and wonderfully made creation, and He knows that you deal daily with pressure coming at you from all sides. He is always present with you, but you may miss His presence because you are so focused on the things that cause your stress.

In John's gospel, we read about a conversation Jesus had with His disciples. Jesus knew that His crucifixion was near and that the way ahead was not going to be easy for those He was leaving behind. In His compassionate way, Jesus was preparing those disciples, telling them that God would send them His Spirit as their Advocate and Comforter. Jesus said to them, and He says to you, "I am leaving you with a gift—peace of mind and heart. And the peace I give is a gift the world cannot give. So don't be troubled or afraid" (John 14:27 NLT).

What a gift! While we cannot slam the door on stress on our path to peace, there are some ways to deal with it. The original Bible word for *spirit* is *pneuma*, and *pneuma* literally means breath or wind. Breathe in His Spirit and His presence today. Those moments when you are focusing on His presence as you take that deep breath will help you find the balance you need to better deal with your stress.

Inhale

"It's not stress that kills us, it is our reaction to it."

(Hans Selye)

"For the Spirit of God has made me, and the breath of the Almighty gives me life"

(Job 33:4 NLT).

"When you inhale, you are taking the strength from God. When you exhale, it represents the service you are giving to the world."

(B. K. S. Iyengar)

Exhale

Dear Father, I ask You to help me experience Your presence. Order my steps, and guide me through all my activities this day. Help me to remember to stop and breathe when I am feeling moments of stress. Help me to remember Your promise and the gift of Your peace. Amen.

Self-Care Steps to Peace

- After you have prayed, continue to sit quietly with your eyes closed. Follow your breath for two minutes, breathing slowly, deeply, through your nose, with abdominal breathing. As you do, imagine that you are inhaling peace and exhaling your stressors.
- At least once during the day when you're feeling stressed, stop what you're doing. Take your pulse, and then follow your breath for two minutes. Inhale for five counts, and exhale for six counts. Then take your pulse again.
- Observe how you are using your phone. Are you turning to it so you will have something to do? Are you checking email and social media constantly in any spare moment?

- How do you feel after scrolling through social media? Do you feel less stressed? More stressed? Renewed? Depressed?
- At your next urge to pick up your phone in an idle moment, pause and take some deep breaths. Take some time to just be present in the moment and notice what you are feeling.
- Designate times to check email and social media so that you are not checking them throughout the day.
- Try deleting social media apps from your phone for a period of time. When you add them back, you may be surprised to find you really have not missed anything.
- Try a *phast* during dinner, during a walk outside, and before bedtime.

Step Two

Moving Away from Stress

"The clearest way into the Universe is
through a forest wilderness."
John Muir

From Dr. Jan

Let's talk about a second pillar of health: movement.
Enjoyable movement can have a positive effect on our
health by distracting us from the stressor and enhancing
our confidence through the achievement of physical
activity. Aerobic exercise—exercise that raises our heart
rate—is good at this. The demand on our body causes us
to focus our mind on the physical effort instead of what
was bothering us. This activity reduces the body's
hormonal response to stress that eventually damages our
organs. It also results in the production of mood—
beneficial neurotransmitters and endorphins. Endorphins
are the body's own chemicals that induce euphoric
feelings and have been previously referred to as a
"runner's high."

You can judge whether your activity is moderate or
vigorous by using the "talk test."[1] During moderate
activity breathing is harder, but you can still easily have a

conversation. Examples include brisk walking or cycling on a flat road. Even gardening, yard work, or active housework can be moderate activity. During vigorous activity you can only say a few or no words before taking a breath. Examples include power walking, jogging, running, swimming, hiking hills, and cycling to include hills.

If moderate or vigorous activity can be done outside, nature can have beneficial effects on our health and well-being and can reduce stress on the body and mind. Many of us can recall that after enjoyable aerobic activity outdoors, such as jogging, cycling, or a brisk walk, we have a different perspective on what was bothering us beforehand.

A formal strategy for getting the benefits of being in nature is the practice of *shinrin-yoku*, or "forest bathing," as started in Japan in the 1980s.[2] This involves a relaxed walk in the forest or in nature—not a brisk hike—that involves intentional mindfulness with use of the senses and sharing what is observed in nature. Studies on forest bathing showed that forest environments lower the level of stress hormone as well as lower the pulse rate and blood pressure. In other words, walking in the forest activates the parasympathetic nervous system—the relaxation response. And you don't even have to be deep in the forest; green spaces in the city can do the same thing.[3]

Many of our urban environments, however, have become devoid of green space. So, what if you don't have access to green space? A study suggests that just looking at an image of trees can provide the same benefits, and smelling an essential oil that comes from trees (such as pine, spruce, frankincense, or elemi) adds to the effect.[4]

And finally, if you don't have an image of trees or an essential oil from trees? Just imagining the sights, sounds, and scents of being outside can activate the relaxation response.

One reason to be active is to counteract insomnia, which is common when we are stressed. Occasional wakefulness at night is normal, especially in times of stress. But we know that thirty percent of adults suffer from insomnia and that it is more common in women and older adults.[5] If insomnia continues for a long time, work and quality of life are affected, and it becomes a significant risk factor for mental illnesses, diabetes, and cardiovascular diseases. Physical activity can be used as a successful treatment to improve sleep quality and decrease the time needed to fall asleep.

There are a number of "sleep hygiene" strategies that can be used as a foundation for healthy sleep.[6]

- Avoid regular physical activity within three hours of bedtime.
- Avoid electronic screens—including television, computer, and cell phone—for at least an hour before bed. Or wear blue-light glasses to filter out the blue light from electronics that inhibits melatonin secretion, a hormone critical for our sleep cycle.
- Stay on a regular schedule for bedtime and waking.

- Limit caffeine intake, especially in the evening. Some people may be more sensitive and need to avoid it in the afternoon and evening.
- Limit alcohol. While alcohol can make it easier to go to sleep, it decreases REM (rapid eye movement) sleep, which is restorative and needed for a healthy sleep cycle.
- Keep the bedroom cool and dark.
- Use the bed only for sleep and sex. If you are wakeful, get up and sit somewhere else to read or do something relaxing until you feel like going to sleep.
- Maintain a healthy diet.

Finally, Dr. Rubin Naiman, a sleep and dream specialist, stated, "Heartfelt prayer is one of the most overlooked strategies for healing insomnia."[7]

Your integrative medicine doctor can recommend some natural supplements for sleep. Essential oils, such as lavender, cedarwood, orange, tangerine, Roman chamomile, and valerian can be very helpful.[8] These can be diffused at the bedside or diluted and made into a roll-on to use on your pillow. (See the steps at the end of this section for instructions.) If you continue to struggle with sleep, talk to your doctor.

From Phyllis

I remember teaching Sunday school to a lively group of eight-year-olds who were learning the creation story and how what God created was good. During activity time, they were given paper and crayons to draw something God had fashioned on the fifth day of creation according to the first chapter of Genesis. I sat at the table and watched zebras, rabbits, birds, fish, and a myriad of other brightly colored animals come almost to life on their papers.

One boy sat quietly staring into space. Then he drew quickly but deliberately two parallel vertical lines almost the length of his paper and followed that with two parallel lines across the top, perpendicular to those two lines. Inside those lines he printed in bold letters *ZOO*. Something tells me that if I had asked Albert to draw what God created on the third day of creation, he would have drawn an identical sign, and he would have written in bold letters *BOTANICAL GARDENS*.

God's choice was to create a perfect garden where the crown of His creation—human beings—would live. He had already created light and water and had separated the heavens from the earth and the waters from dry land. The Bible says, "Then the LORD God planted a garden in Eden in the east, and there he placed the man he had made. The LORD God made all sorts of trees grow up from the ground—trees that were beautiful and that produced delicious fruit" (Genesis 2:8–9 NLT).

Can you imagine the forest and vegetation that grew in that perfect garden watered by the springs bubbling from the earth? Think of God's imagination in creating the giant sequoias, the noble oaks, the deep-rooted pines, the prickly cactus, and the velvety lamb's ear. Then think of all the blossoms—the delicate orchid, fragrant rose, sweet gardenias, and the moonflower. And to think so many of these have medicinal properties, and God gave all of this to us.

The Bible tells us that Jesus often withdrew early in the day and went alone to a garden to pray. We read in the gospel accounts of how Jesus crossed the Kidron Valley with His disciples and went to the garden to pray on the night He was arrested. I had the great and humbling experience of walking around the Mount of Olives and seeing the gnarled and twisted trees that many believe were the very trees Jesus knelt under to pray. I have tried to imagine what those hours and days were like for Him. He was human as well as divine, and He felt every stress that you and I could ever feel. And when He was the most stressed, Jesus felt the need to be alone in the garden to talk to His Father.

When my husband, Bill, was diagnosed with cancer, we inquired of his doctors what we could do to keep him the healthiest during weeks of chemotherapy prior to his surgery and his recovery after the removal of his kidney. His primary-care physician, oncologist, and surgeon almost in unison instructed him to move—to walk, preferably outdoors as his strength and the weather permitted. Prior to his diagnosis, Bill was accustomed to daily long walks and hikes in the hills. During treatment and recovery, some days he could only walk a short way on level ground, but he kept at it. His walks grew longer and more challenging as his strength returned and we hiked the hills again. We followed his doctors' advice, and I can tell you it was so beneficial to his convalescence and to his general well-being—and mine, too, as his caregiver.

We have the great pleasure of continuing to walk together for a couple of miles almost every morning under a canopy of trees and surrounded by the vegetation that grows in the Texas Hill Country. I breathe the air and watch the ever-changing landscape after a rain or when the leaves are beginning to change color or when they're laden with frost. Sometimes we talk, and sometimes we are quiet with our own thoughts. Either way, the walk is energizing and relaxing. Be assured that wading in the creek or picking up a heart-shaped rock or looking for the vermillion flycatcher in his favorite oak are not just activities for children.

Maybe it's our longing for Eden, for the indescribable place God created for us, but being close to nature is therapeutic and helps us gain a new perspective. If you can, find a place to walk under the trees today. But even if you must only imagine it, close your eyes, picture it, and breathe deeply of His spirit as you walk.

Inhale

"I will plant trees in the barren desert—
cedar, acacia, myrtle, olive, cypress, fir, and pine.
I am doing this so all who see this miracle
will understand what it means—
that it is the LORD who has done this,
the Holy One of Israel who created it." (Isaiah 41:19–
20 NLT)

"I took a walk in the woods and came out taller than the trees."

(Henry David Thoreau)

"Reading about nature is fine, but if a person walks in the woods and listens carefully, he can learn more than what is in books, for they speak with the voice of God."

(George Washington Carver)

Exhale

Dear Father, thank You for giving us such a beautiful world. Thank you that when I look upon it, I am drawn closer to You as I am reminded of Your creativity, Your greatness, and Your attention to detail. Amen.

Self-Care Steps to Peace

- Think about how much time you spend outdoors compared to time looking at a digital screen (phone, computer, TV). Do the best you can to log your screen time for just one normal day. Determine to decrease that time and increase your time outdoors.

- If you enjoy vigorous exercise such as running or cycling, work this into your schedule when you are feeling stressed. (Check with your doctor before beginning any new exercise program.) When you can, make use of the outdoors to get the benefits of sunshine and being in nature.

- If more moderate exercise is for you, take a brisk walk outdoors. Go a little farther than you usually do.

- At a separate time from when you do vigorous or moderate exercise, take time for a slow walk in a green space, and activate your senses. Notice the sounds of birds, the breeze, your footsteps on the ground. Do some deep breathing through your nose and notice the smells. Do you smell the trees? The grass? Feel the warmth of the sunshine, the coolness of a breeze, or the chill of a winter wind. As you walk, give God thanks for His gifts of nature.

- If you are having difficulty sleeping, review the sleep hygiene strategies noted earlier in this section. Use essential oils that support sleep in an ultrasonic diffuser at your bedside, or make a roll-on using essential oils to use on your pillow. Try putting ten drops of lavender, five drops of cedarwood, and five drops of orange in a ten-ml roll-on bottle. (See Self-Care Resources for where to find roll-on bottles.) Fill to the top with a carrier oil such as almond oil or fractionated coconut oil. Roll the blend onto your pillow.

Step Three

Stress Eating

"Every day brings a choice:
To practice stress or to practice peace."
Joan Borysenko

From Dr. Jan

This section will focus on what you're eating and how that is affected by stress. Check in with what and how you are eating and ask if your eating habits could be directly related to stress. While stress decreases appetite acutely due to the effects of adrenaline, cortisol continues to be released with long-term stress and can lead to increased appetite and weight gain.

In addition, we tend to favor foods high in sugar and/or fat when stressed. In particular, we tend to crave "comfort" foods that satisfy cravings and make us feel better in the short-term by increasing blood-sugar levels quickly. However, this leads to the release of a spike of insulin, which acts to store glucose and causes blood-sugar levels to crash. The brain and body then feel deprived, and cravings start again.

Carbohydrates have been categorized as simple or complex as a way to describe their absorption and effect on blood sugar, but a more accurate way to determine the rate at which carbohydrate foods increase the blood-sugar level is measured by the glycemic index.[1] This is a scale of one to one hundred that measures how quickly carbohydrates are metabolized and enter the blood-stream as blood sugar. A rating of one hundred is the maximum rating, meaning that these foods are turned into blood sugar most quickly. Examples of high glyce-mic-index foods include those containing large amounts of refined sugar or high fructose corn syrup, such as cakes, cookies, sweetened beverages, sports drinks, or processed high-carbohydrate foods such as potato chips and crackers. In general, foods with a glycemic index of seventy and above are digested and absorbed quickly.

One way to stop the cycle of cravings is to eat lower glycemic-index foods. These are foods that take longer to digest and/or contain fiber. These are absorbed and turned into blood sugar more slowly. Examples are berries, apples, pears, whole grains, chickpeas, sweet potatoes, and oatmeal (non-instant). A rating of fifty-five and lower is considered a low glycemic index, and these stabilize blood sugar. A rating between fifty-five and seventy is considered moderate. These can still be satisfying but do not cause the blood sugar spike and subsequent spike of insulin that high glycemic-index foods do. You can check the ratings of your favorite foods at https://glycemicindex.com and other sites. You may already know what effect foods with high refined sugar content have on you.

Another advantage foods such as fruits, vegetables, and whole grains have is that they supply other beneficial nutrients such as vitamins, minerals, polyphenols, antioxidants, and fiber. Foods high in fiber help to balance blood sugar and avoid insulin surges. Examples of high-fiber foods include whole grains, beans, leafy greens, berries, and nuts. Watch the amount of nuts since they are calorie dense. A small handful is usually a reasonable serving.

One concept of choosing healthy food is to "eat the rainbow." In other words, choose natural foods of many colors to include a variety of phytonutrients—nutrients produced by plants—in your diet. (Processed foods with artificial food colorings don't count!) Dark leafy greens like spinach or kale and berries will help with this goal. The leafy greens and nuts are good sources of magnesium, which helps to calm the autonomic nervous system and relieve psychological stress.

Take a break for some tea. Choose an herbal tea like chamomile, peppermint, or lemon balm. Going through the ceremony of making a cup of tea and then drinking it slowly, savoring the taste, can be calming.

Mindful eating is a useful practice to develop a more conscious relationship to food, especially in times of stress.[2] While we *know* we should only eat when hungry and stop eating when we are full, in our society, where food is plentiful and where we've been taught to "Clean your plate," we forget what this feels like. Before eating, take a moment to be mindful and aware of whether you are actually hungry. Are you reaching for food because you are stressed? Thirsty? Anxious? If you are not hungry, try drinking some water and then doing something else—taking a walk, reading a book, meditating.

When you are hungry, savor each bite of food. What are you tasting? Can you identify if it is sweet, salty, sour, savory, or bitter? What is the texture of the food? Put your fork down between each bite. After several minutes of eating, take a break for a couple of minutes. This helps allow your brain to catch up with your stomach and detect when you are getting full, and you can learn to stop eating before becoming too full.

You don't always have choices about the stress you're experiencing, but you do have choices about how you feed your feelings. Don't let your stress put you on the roller coaster of sugar highs and lows. Make choices that will make you healthier in the long run.

From Phyllis

God designed our bodies to need fuel—the right kind of fuel that He provides. Since consuming food is something that every human must do to live, eating is not a bad habit that we can just give up. Making wise choices about food and food preparation therefore become critical to living healthy lives. Making those choices require time, commitment, and educating ourselves—just a few more things to do! For many of us who are not only responsible for our own choices but also for our family members, food planning and preparation can add more stress to our already hurried lives. One of my favorite stories from the Bible is about nourishment for the body and nourishment for the soul. Perhaps there is a lesson for us in this story.

Did you grow up with the old adage, "Idle hands are the devil's workshop"? I did. And the way Mama quoted it, I thought it came straight from the Bible. Sounded like a Proverb to me and believing it has kept me busy all my life. Although there are some instructive Bible passages about the danger of idleness, this is not one of them. People who research idioms traced this one back to Chaucer.

Living with responsibilities and the fear of idle hands can create opportunities for major stress. It can keep you busy when you really should be intentionally idle. The Bible story of the two sisters, Mary and Martha, illustrates this point. I find it interesting that it is Doctor Luke who tells us this story about Martha's stress (see Luke 10).

Jesus and His disciples were in Bethany, a small village outside Jerusalem. As was her custom, Martha offered hospitality to them. Can you imagine her stress when she realized she had a house full of hungry men to feed? No local takeout. No microwave. No preparations made. And to make matters worse, her sister Mary, who was supposed to be helping, was sitting at Jesus' feet listening to His every word. Both sisters were focused, but they were focused on entirely different things.

Perhaps steam was coming from both her ears when Martha left the kitchen, stomped (my interpretation) into the room where all of them sat, and literally scolded

Jesus, telling Him He should instruct Mary to help her with the preparations. In modern-day language, Jesus might have said, "Martha, you're getting all stressed out. You need to take a breath, or maybe you should take a walk." But He responded gently and firmly, "My dear Martha, you are worried and upset over all these details! There is only one thing worth being concerned about. Mary has discovered it, and it will not be taken away from her" (Luke 10:41–42 NLT). Turns out what Martha thought was Mary's idleness wasn't idleness at all.

Chances are if you're stressed, you're really identifying with Martha in this story. The good news is that you don't have to be Martha all the time. You don't even have to choose between being Martha or Mary. There is no need for being "either or." One is not right and the other wrong. There is simply the right time for being either. Notice Jesus was aware of Martha's stress and did not tell Martha what she was doing was unimportant. He just reminded her not to be so worried and upset about it.

There are times when we need to be Martha, fulfilling our responsibilities, even if they seem overwhelming and pile more stress on us. But like Mary, we must take the time to feed our spirits on God's Word, to pray, to be still and listen, and to reflect. Sometimes our best work is being still, focusing on priorities, getting in touch with what is causing our stress, and just relaxing in God's presence. When we take this kind of time for ourselves, then we are likely more ready to be Martha and get busy again. Be busy, but take time to be still.

It is not easy being Mary when the world requires us to be Martha. Moving from stress to peace and deciding when to be Martha and when to be Mary are conscious choices. When you feel the stress and long for peace, fold your intentionally idle hands, place them in your lap, breathe deeply, and pray, asking God to help you find the balance.

Inhale

"There is no trouble so great or grave that cannot be much diminished by a nice cup of tea."

(Bernard-Paul Heroux)

"Don't worry about anything; instead, pray about everything. Tell God what you need, and thank him for all he has done. Then you will experience God's peace, which exceeds anything we can understand. His peace will guard your hearts and minds as you live in Christ Jesus."

(Philippians 4:6–7 NLT)

"In the rush and noise of life, as you have intervals, step home within yourselves and be still. Wait upon God, and feel His good presence; this will carry you evenly through your day's business."

(William Penn)

Exhale

Pray: Father, in my busyness, help me to be intentional about finding time to be quiet and sense your Presence. Help me find balance in work, play, and rest, and help me to choose the best foods to nourish my body so that it will function as You designed it. Thank You that You invite me to sit at Your feet and be still before You. Amen.

Self-Care Steps to Peace

- Before you eat, stop, and think about whether you are really hungry. If it is not mealtime, try drinking some water first.

- If you are eating because you are stressed or anxious, try doing something else first. Take a walk or read or journal.

- Think about the way you snack. Instead of grabbing cookies or chips, reach for some apple slices with almond butter, carrots or celery with hummus, berries with yogurt, or a small handful of nuts.

- Add some dark, leafy greens to one of your meals. See if you don't feel better and if this helps break you from the stress-eating cycle.

- Buy an assortment of herbal teas you'd like to try. Include chamomile, lemon, and peppermint. Use your favorite teacup, and make this an enjoyable ritual, a time just for yourself. As the tea steeps, enjoy a few moments of deep breathing as you inhale the fragrance of the tea.

Step Four

Spirit Connections

"We cultivate love when we allow our most
vulnerable and powerful selves to be deeply seen
and known, and when we honor the spiritual
connection that grows from that offering with
trust, respect, kindness, and affection."

Brené Brown

From Dr. Jan

One of the reasons we experience stress is that things
happen to us that we can't control. We can use our spirit
to accept things we cannot control and change our
response to them. This action empowers us again and
allows us to control our response, even if we can't control
our circumstances.

Contact and discussion with other people can often
help us put into perspective the problem causing our
stress. We may be inclined to bury a problem within and
not discuss it, but telling someone else about it may
actually help us gain some insights to controlling our
response, even as we explain it to someone else. A spouse
or family member may be the most accessible, but at
times we need a "third voice" who is not as close to the

situation. Many times, a friend, a minister, or a rabbi can serve in this role. In times of severe stress, talk to a mental health professional.

In explaining the situation to a listening ear, several things can happen. First, we may realize that things are not as bad as we thought. Second, we can better discern the problem that is causing us stress. Third, we—or the person we are talking to—can recognize solutions we have not thought about before. In fact, we may realize there are actions that we must take. Finally, when situations are indeed serious and do not seem to have a solution, it can make us feel better just to have a sympathetic ear. This connection of our spirit with someone else's spirit can be very therapeutic.

There will be times when we have situations we cannot share with others. Discussion with a mental health professional is useful here. Also, at those times, it can be helpful to write down our thoughts. This can be a clarifying exercise. I would recommend manually writing by hand instead of typing on the computer. There is something about spilling out thoughts out on the page that helps us think more clearly. This exercise can also help us let go of things we can't control. Again, we may realize actions that must be taken or identify how we can respond differently. This is our spirit at work.

From Phyllis

Words matter. They can bring hope and healing, or they can bring pain and sorrow. Words matter when you speak them to someone else, and they especially matter when you speak them to yourself.

In the English language, verbs are words we use to describe an action or a state of being. Picture this: I *walked* alongside the stream in the forest, and I *felt* the cool morning breeze in my face. That sentence describes an action and a feeling. And since English verbs have tenses that speak to the time element, we can talk about our past or what is going on in our lives right this moment or what we hope or plan for the future.

Are you aware that there are seven thousand languages in the world, and some of them have no way of communicating a future tense? For instance, for people who speak Mandarin Chinese, the present and future are the same. Can you imagine thinking of present time and future time as the same? I find it impossible to think about life without a distinction between the two. And yet for many people, this is how they perceive and record their lives, and it affects them in profound ways. According to Keith Chen, a behavioral economist, futureless languages can even affect the saving and spending habits of their speakers because language affects the way they think.[1]

If futureless languages can affect world economies, then just imagine the power the words you read or speak have over your thoughts, attitudes, and even responses to stress.

God created human beings for relationship— relationship with Him and with other human beings— and we use language to build and maintain those relationships. As Dr. Jan mentioned, conversations with trusted family members or friends can be helpful when we are feeling stress. Verbalizing our feelings to someone we trust is often cathartic, but it can also be difficult.

Writing down what you are feeling often helps you clarify your thoughts. Journaling is a way to record your life, your feelings, your thoughts, and your reflections, and it can be effective in helping you cope with stress. I have found that journaling can also be a helpful tool in decision-making. Oh, the things I have learned about myself as I have read back through my journals of past years.

But the most important thing I write down daily is Scripture. When I started the discipline of Scripture writing as a part of my daily devotional life, I realized I was doing more than just copying verses. I had images of birds scratching in the grass and soil for seeds and kernels, and that was exactly what I was doing— searching for a kernel of truth or a seed of hope. And since "scratching" is what some call their handwriting, thus the phrase "Scripture Scratching" was born and became the title of journals my husband and I created.[2]

As I copy a verse from Scripture, I meditate, asking what the text is saying specifically to me and my present circumstances. Then I pray, asking God to help me apply the verse to the way I live my life this day. I find that the passage will come back into my thoughts throughout the day, and often I even have opportunity to share it with someone else.

In his book of wisdom, Solomon said of words, "Tie them on your fingers as a reminder. Write them deep within your heart" (Proverbs 7:3 NLT). Words matter because words shape our thoughts, and our thoughts influence our actions. Imagine how putting comforting or encouraging Scripture verses into your mind will influence your thinking today and in the future.

Inhale

"When I was upset and beside myself, you calmed me down and cheered me up."

(Psalm 94:19 MSG)

"Writing is a spiritual practice in that people that have no spiritual path can undertake it and, as they write, they begin to wake up to a larger connection. After a while people tend to find that there is some muse that they are connecting to."

(Julia Cameron)

"I can shake off everything as I write, my sorrows disappear and my courage is reborn."

(Anne Frank)

Exhale

God give me the serenity to accept things which cannot
be changed;
Give me the courage to change things which must be
changed;

And the wisdom to distinguish one from the other.
(Attributed to Reinhold Niebuhr and others)

Self-Care Steps to Peace

- Talk to a trusted friend about your source of stress. As you speak, listen to yourself and your friend for more insights and discernment.
- Try writing about your stress—its sources, how you respond, your ideas for dealing with the stress. You can also visualize letting go of the things you cannot control as you are writing.
- Talk or write about your response to the situation and how that is causing you stress about the future.
- As you write, practice Phyllis's Scripture Scratching. Write down Psalm 94:19 and Philippians 4:6–7 today.

Step Five

Putting Self-Care Steps to Peace into Practice

"Almost everything will work again if you unplug
it for a few minutes…including you."

Anne Lamott

From Dr. Jan

We've written about deep breathing, moderate and vigorous activity, walking outdoors, stabilizing blood sugar with healthy eating, and spiritual connections with friends and with writing. We are using these four pillars of self-care—breath, movement, healthy eating, and spiritual connection—as strategies to seek peace instead of stress.

Now it is time to integrate these strategies into your routine. We talked in Step One about intentional breathing and using slow, deep breaths to counteract chronic stress. Think about using intentional breathing throughout the day. At several times during your daily routine, take a minute to check in with your breath. You can do this while you are in the car commuting to or from work or when you are preparing for a meal.

Evaluate your breathing. Is it shallow, rapid, noisy, irregular? Is the breath just from your chest? Are you inhaling through your mouth? Take this opportunity to breathe deeply and slowly. Inhale through your nose and use abdominal breathing. By checking in regularly throughout the day, healthier breathing can become a habit. We will learn some other breathing techniques in the next sections, but the simple step of learning to take slow, deep breaths routinely during the day will keep you healthier.

In Step Two, we talked about movement and the power of aerobic activity in distracting us from our stressors. There is further benefit in decreasing stress if we can do this outside in nature. If running or cycling is not for you, even a brisk walk outdoors is an excellent strategy for mitigating stress. You've thought about how much time you spend in front of a digital screen compared to how much time you spend outdoors or in enjoyable movement. How will you incorporate outdoor time into your schedule? Morning works better for some people, and afternoon or early evening works better for others. Vigorous exercise within three hours of bedtime is not recommended because it can be detrimental to falling asleep. Find what time of day works best for you, and try daily enjoyable movement for a week to see if you are less stressed.

The practice of forest bathing, or forest therapy, is a mindful and unrushed encounter with the outdoors. The primary intent here is not exercise but to connect with nature using all of our senses—sight, sound, smell, taste, and touch. Take a leisurely, mindful walk outdoors, and notice the sights around you, the smell of the trees and

the grass, the feel of the bark on the trees and the coolness of the grass. Walk slowly, sit, or stand still and
notice what is in motion. Share with others or in a journal
what you experienced. There are guides that are formally
trained in the practice of forest therapy and you can learn
more about it at the Association of Nature and Forest
Therapy Guides and Programs.[1] Dr. Susan Bartlett
Hackenmiller, an integrative medicine physician, has
written an outdoor adventurer's guide to forest bathing
that will be very helpful in seriously pursuing this
practice.[2]

Step Three addressed stress eating. It's a habit many
of us have, and it takes recognition of it and calling it
exactly that to start shifting the habit. Changing eating
habits is difficult. It can even mean revising our grocery
lists and finding time to prepare something healthy.
Stress eating often occurs between meals at snack times,
so it helps to have healthier snacks readily available so
we don't choose candy, chips, or cookies. Take some time
weekly to slice vegetables and individually package them
and to have some fruit snacks ready; this makes it easier
to make a healthy choice. After a while, it becomes a
habit, and these become the snacks of choice. To add
dark, leafy greens to some of your meals, try Dr. Weil's
Tuscan Kale Salad recipe.[3] This is an easy and delicious
way to add super nutrients to your food.

Spirit connection is from Step Four. It also takes time
and intention to connect with others and with our spirit.
Set aside some time to discuss what is causing you stress
with a trusted friend, spiritual mentor, or mental health

professional. It can also be helpful to write down your stressors. This can identify and clarify problems, which leads to solutions or at least changing the way we think about them.

Perhaps most important, a practice of mindfulness is needed to integrate these strategies. Jon Kabat-Zinn, the founder of Mindfulness-Based Stress Reduction, defines *mindfulness* as "awareness that arises through paying attention, on purpose, in the present moment, non-judgmentally."[4] We are used to always having a distraction—our mobile phone, TV, radio in the car, talking to someone, something to read. Practicing mindfulness is especially helpful for connecting to our spirit. We talked about following the breath in Step One. Take some time to follow your breath and let go of your thoughts. Just concentrate on your breathing. Thoughts from what happened yesterday, what we need to do today, and what we can worry about will pop into our minds. When they do, it is not a failure of our mindfulness; in fact, we are observing what is happening with our thoughts in the present, which is mindfulness. Just say, "Okay," observe those thoughts, and turn back to your breath.

Dr. Herbert Benson described the relaxation response in the Western medical literature in 1974.[5] He noted four elements to elicit the response:

- mental device: a stimulus such as a repetitive sound, spoken or unspoken
- passive attitude: disregard of distracting thoughts
- decreased muscle tone: a comfortable posture

- quiet environment: a quiet room or place of worship with eyes closed

He cited several examples in historical Judeo-Christian culture of levels of spiritual attainment for closer unity with God that use these basic tenets and noted that they have in common the physiologic changes that can occur in deep meditation.

In Step One we started with two minutes of following the breath. See if you can increase by a minute a day until you've worked up to at least five minutes. Taking this time to clear our minds can help make the decisions we have during the day easier and help to counteract stress. Mindfulness can decrease stress and its unhealthy effects, including high blood pressure.

From Phyllis

It's not always easy to be mindful in a Martha world. Often, we do not even want to deal with the present, let alone be mindful of it, when responsibilities are torturing us and people are pulling at us and the clock is ticking and our list is growing longer. I need a deep breath just writing these words.

A look at Jesus gives us a perfect model of mindfulness. In Jesus' humanity, He experienced serious stress. He was continually surrounded by people, most often by His disciples but sometimes by large, curious crowds. Many were critical of Him and misunderstood Him, and He was under continual scrutiny by the religious leaders of His day. He rarely had any time for Himself unless He intentionally withdrew from those around Him early in the day to pray. We can only imagine the weight of responsibility He must have felt.

Yet Scripture reveals to us that He was a man of peace. There was a calmness about Him that attracted people. He never seemed to be in a hurry, and He was always mindful of others and the situation, even in a crowd.

One day as He was being questioned by a group of people, one of the leaders of the synagogue approached Jesus. The man was distraught because his daughter had just died. He begged Jesus to come and bring the girl back to life, so Jesus and His disciples followed the man down the busy streets of the village to his home. As Jesus was on His way, He sensed that someone had touched His robe. Even on His way to raise a girl from the dead, Jesus turned to the ailing woman and healed her (see Matthew 9).

Jesus could maintain peace under enormous pressure because He knew who He was, what His ultimate purpose was, and how that purpose guided His daily activities. Jesus also asked people to help Him get His job done. He would often lead His disciples into the mountains or the desert just to rest and refuel. And most important, Jesus had a practice of withdrawing from others and finding a solitary place to pray. Jesus was mindful of who He was, of His needs, and of the needs of others.

Perhaps being mindful of who you truly are, what your ultimate purpose is, and who you're ultimately attempting to please would help you to be calm in stressful times. To do that, like Jesus, find a restful place to relax and refuel, and follow Him to a solitary place to pray on your way to finding peace.

Inhale

"Now may the Lord of peace himself give you his peace at all times and in every situation. The Lord be with you all."

(2 Thessalonians 3:16 NLT)

"How we pay attention to the present moment largely determines the character of our experience, and therefore, the quality of our lives."

(Sam Harris)

Exhale

Dear God, thank You that when I ask for peace, You give me Your presence. Help me to learn to deal with the stresses of life and take care of my body, which You made with such detail. I ask that You make me mindful of You and mindful of myself in the circumstances of my life, and to remind me to care for myself as You care for me. Amen.

Self-Care Steps to Peace

- Remember to breathe—deeply and slowly—throughout your day.

- Use regular moderate or vigorous activity to de-stress if you enjoy that movement.

- Take a walk, preferably where you can experience nature.

- Feed your body, not your stress.

- If you are between meals, pause before you eat to determine why you want to eat. If you are not hungry, do something else—walk, play with the dog, read, meditate.

- Talk to a trusted family member, friend, or mental health professional about your stress.

- Write your thoughts about your stress and how you plan to deal with it.

- Write something encouraging from God's Word each day. The Scripture Scratching guide is free and covers topics such as gratitude, hope, joy, peace, and patience.[6]

- Be mindful as you take care of your soul, your whole self.

Part Two

Self-Care for Anxiety

Step One

The Perfect Breath

"If you want to conquer the anxiety of life, live in
the moment, live in the breath."

Amit Ray

From Dr. Jan

We all experience anxiety from time to time. However,
anxiety can become more than just a passing feeling. It
can be disabling and cause emotional as well as physical
symptoms, resulting in an anxiety disorder. It is estimated that forty million adults, or eighteen percent of adults
in the US, have an anxiety disorder at any given time.[1]
Anxiety is feeling fearful, worried, or nervous about a
situation. Anxiety is often a result of stress, but there are
many potential risk factors such as difficult life events,
genetics, and biochemical changes in the brain. While
some anxiety can be useful in getting us prepared to
perform at our best for a presentation or an athletic
event, when anxiety becomes excessive, it can be disabling.

In the previous section, we talked about dealing with
stressors so that chronic stress can be avoided. However,
anxiety may already be present as a result of chronic

stress. And sometimes, anxiety is present even without identifiable stressors. Some types of anxiety that are severe and chronic are classified as disorders, such as generalized anxiety disorder, obsessive compulsive disorder, panic disorder, acute stress disorder, and phobias.[2] These types of disorders may require medication such as anxiolytics (anti-anxiety medications) or anti-depressants, and persons with these disorders should seek care from a medical professional. Psychotherapy with a mental-health professional can also be helpful, and your doctor can guide you when this is needed.

Anxiolytic medications, such as benzodiazepines (benzos) may be needed for some of the aforementioned conditions. Examples are alprazolam (Xanax), lorazepam (Ativan), and diazepam (Valium). Benzos, however, may be overused and are often prescribed chronically instead of for a short period of time. These are some of the most commonly used medications in the US.[3] These medications act on the brain to cause sedation and increase the effect of a calming neurotransmitter, GABA (gamma-aminobutyric acid). Side effects include drowsiness, dizziness, confusion, weakness, abnormal sleep, nausea, and depression. Moreover, benzo use leads to physical dependence. Over time, the dose often has to be increased to have the desired effect, and stopping the dose suddenly causes rebound symptoms. People are often not aware of the side effects and dependence problems related to these medications. After chronic use of these agents, discontinuation must be done gradually and under medical supervision.[4]

So there are good reasons to seek complementary approaches to anxiety, and there are self-care techniques that can help.[5] These techniques can be integrated with medications and/or psychotherapy if those are needed. One of the complementary approaches to anxiety is intentional breathing.[6] In the previous section we talked about breathing slowly and deeply through the nose and using the abdomen. This is a good way to start self-care when feeling stressed or anxious.

As an extension of the slow, deep, abdominal breathing we discussed, Drs. Brown and Gerbarg have described a simple method in their book *The Healing Power of Breath*.[7] The method is Coherent Breathing, a technique that slows breathing to about five to six breaths per minute. They recommend closing the eyes, relaxing the hands, inhaling to a slow count of four and exhaling to a slow count of four while breathing through the nose. This is easy to practice with their accessible soundtrack using chimes (see Self-Care Resources). The practice can be done for five to ten minutes initially, working up to twenty minutes.

In James Nestor's well-researched book *Breath*, he describes the perfect breath at rest as 5.5 breaths per minute, with a 5.5 second inhale and a 5.5 second exhale.[8] Interestingly, this results in taking in 5.5 liters of air per minute. This pattern and rate have been used by those studying breathing techniques for medicine and athletic performance over many years, as well as those who have studied patterns of both Western and Eastern religious traditional prayers. Indeed, anxiety is not the only reason to slow our breath rate; it appears to be good for our overall health.

There are other specific breathing techniques that are steps to relaxation and calming, and one is the "4-7-8 breath" made famous by Dr. Andrew Weil of the Andrew Weil Center for Integrative Medicine at University of Arizona.[9] To do this relaxation exercise, sit with a straight back. Place the tip of your tongue right behind your upper front teeth and keep it there during the exercise. When you exhale through your mouth, you will exhale around your tongue in this position. To begin the breath, inhale through your nose quietly to a count of four. Hold your breath for seven counts. Then exhale through your mouth, with a "whoosh" sound, to a count of eight. Each count does not need to be one second; it is the ratio that is important. As you get used to doing the exercise, you will be able to slow down the count.

As you first do the exercise, do no more than four of the 4-7-8 breaths at a time. After a month of practice, you should be able to do eight breaths at a time. Do a set of four 4-7-8 breaths at least twice daily. Use it when you feel stressed—and try to do it before you react to the stressor. Use it when you feel anxious. You can also use it to help you unwind and fall asleep. Slowing the breath and the short hold of the inhaled breath activates your parasympathetic nervous system—your relaxation response—which is very powerful. This relaxation exercise increases in effectiveness over time as you practice it.

From Phyllis

I remember vividly a mid-September morning as my husband and I stood together atop a mountain near Vail, Colorado. We had hiked for more than an hour up Knob Hill Trail to get to the summit. It wasn't the climb or the altitude that took my breath away. It was the sheer joy and beauty of the experience and looking at the valley below and the 360-degree panorama of mountains shimmering with the gold of aspens. Those are the kinds of moments that we yearn for—those beautiful moments that take your breath away.

Our worries and fears can also take our breath away—those moments when anxiety puts our chests in a vise and we feel the suffocation of severe stress. We experience anxiety because we are afraid—afraid of losing someone we love, of losing our health, of losing a job, of not being able to pay the bills... The list of things we fear losing goes on. But all our fears are related to the feeling of loss of control. We desperately want to be in control so things go the way we want them to go—as though we could really control that.

I remember another scene, this time from my child-hood. Maybe you can relate to this. Confessionally, I was a willful child who liked to have my way. I was about four years old, and I was having myself an award-winning tantrum because I hadn't gotten what I wanted.

Another way of saying this is that is I was not in control of my situation. I cried and sobbed and cried some more and finally refused to breathe. As I began to turn blue, I remember my mother taking my shoulders, getting in my face, and calmly telling me to breathe.

The book of Job tells us the story of a wealthy man of good character and strong faith. In the story, we learn that Job was stripped of his wealth, his servants, his children, and finally his health. He lost everything, including all control over his life and circumstances. Three of his friends showed up to grieve with him and offered their opinions as to why he was suffering so. Sitting in his mess, Job was at one point so distraught that he even cursed the day he was born.

But Job did not trust his feelings, and his story doesn't end there. In the end, Job had a most enlightening conversation with God where he learned once again that God, the Maker of all there is, has infinite power and is ultimately in control. Job accepted the constraint of his own limited understanding and trusted God completely. And for Job, God returned to him all that he had lost.

Most of us will not experience the catastrophic losses Job did, yet we feel the anxiety, the fear of loss, and our own inadequate skills to cope. And most of us will never have the kind of conversation with God that Job had, but the good news is that God does speak to us about our fears and anxieties.

Matthew reminded us of the futility of being anxious when he asked the question, "Can all your worries add a single moment to your life?" (Matthew 6:27 NLT). God wants us to trust Him as Job did, to trust that He is ultimately in control. God wants us to breathe freely, deeply, and without fear—so much so that the phrase "Fear not" occurs more than one hundred times in the Bible.

About my mountaintop experience in Colorado—the one that took my breath away. That was one year after my husband was diagnosed with a life-threatening cancer followed by months of chemotherapy and surgery. There were more anxious moments, hours, and days during that year than I care to remember. What I do choose to remember and hang on to is that in times when God did not remove the circumstances that caused me to feel anxious, His Spirit was present reminding me to breathe and to trust Him.

I won't tell you not to be anxious. Who can live in this Age of Anxiety without feeling some degree of anxiousness? But I do offer you a word of encouragement: you are not alone in your fears. You may feel alone, but be like Job and don't trust your feelings. Trust the One who made and loves you. Hang on, breathe deeply, and ask God to make His presence known to you.

Inhale

"This is my command—be strong and courageous! Do not be afraid or discouraged. For the LORD your God is with you wherever you go."

(Joshua 1:9 NLT)

"Cast all your anxiety upon him because he cares for you."

(1 Peter 5:7 NIV)

Exhale

Father, there are times when I feel I cannot breathe from the stress and anxiety. Help me to remember that I am not alone and that You are present with me in every circumstance. Give me courage to do the things I need to do to take care of myself. Amen.

Self-Care Steps to Calm

- Take five minutes at the beginning or end of your day to practice Coherent Breathing. Close your eyes, relax your hands, and breath through your nose. Inhale for a slow count of four; exhale for a slow count of four. The inhale plus the exhale is one breath. Check to see if you are breathing about five to six times a minute.

- During the day, when you feel stressed or anxious, stop and practice the 4-7-8 breath relaxation exercise. Inhale through your nose for four counts and hold your breath for seven counts. Then exhale through your mouth with a "whoosh" for eight counts. Do a total of four of these breaths. See if you are thinking more clearly and can make a better decision after this exercise.

- Remember, you are not alone in your fears and anxiety. God is always near. As you're taking a deep, relaxing breath, close your eyes and recall one beautiful moment in your life. Picture all the details, including the scenery, the people who were there, the weather, and the sounds. Imagine that you feel that way again.

Step Two

Physical Activity Can Reduce Anxiety

"If you can't fly then run, if you can't run then
walk, if you can't walk then crawl, but whatever
you do you have to keep moving forward."
Martin Luther King Jr.

Dr. Jan

It is estimated that as many as forty percent of persons
treated for anxiety will relapse within the first year after
stopping treatment.[1] Professional medical assessment is
needed to determine when medications are needed and
how long they should be given. Whether or not medications are needed, integrative therapies add some tools to
the toolbox for combatting anxiety. Intentional breathing
as discussed in Step One is an effective intervention for
many. What are other self-care interventions for individuals with anxiety?

There is increasing evidence that lifestyle interventions including physical activity are an effective part of
reducing anxiety symptoms. Movement meditation
activities such as yoga, tai chi, and qi gong can be
effective, and may be especially beneficial for those who
cannot tolerate vigorous aerobic activity, such as jogging

or swimming.[2] Yoga has been shown to increase GABA, that calming neurotransmitter.[3]

And *pranayama*, the breath-control practice that is used in yoga, is like the intentional breathing practices that activate the parasympathetic, or relaxation, response. Yoga and these movement meditation activities are generally safe, and serious injuries are rare.[4] We have added information in the Self-Care Resources section for you to learn more about movement meditations.

The Centers for Disease Control and Prevention recommend 150 minutes of moderate-intensity or seventy-five minutes of vigorous-intensity aerobic activity weekly.[5] Moderate activity would include brisk walking, gardening, or cycling on flat roads. Examples of vigorous activity include running, cycling on hills, swimming, and power walking. Muscle-strengthening activity such as weight training, push-ups or some types of yoga is recommended twice weekly. The activity can be spread out over the week. So, for instance, 150 minutes of moderate activity could be thirty minutes a day for five days a week. A recent review showed benefit for moderate to vigorous aerobic activity for people with anxiety and formally diagnosed anxiety disorders.[6]

Western medicine has advanced in the recognition of Eastern practices such as the movement meditations of yoga, tai chi, and qi gong, as previously mentioned. Some Traditional Chinese Medicine (TCM) practices such as acupuncture are also recognized as helpful. Studies have shown acupuncture can be beneficial for pain, anxiety, insomnia, and more. So, it is worth reviewing

TCM to see what we can learn from it. Ancient scripts about TCM describe paradigms still used today. TCM refers to qi (chi) as the energy in the body. Acupuncture uses the meridian system, a series of energy channels throughout the body and named for organs in the body, to balance qi and thereby address imbalances that result in disease.[7]

TCM describes three energy centers in the body called the *dan tiens*. The lower dan tien, in the lower abdominal area, regulates the overall energy in the body. The middle dan tien oversees the heart, thymus, throat, and the emotional body. The upper dan tien involves the brain, head, and spiritual body. The three centers interact with each other and the meridians to influence the body's energy. The lower dan tien connects us to the earth's energy field and is vital to staying creative and support-ed. We often need to "ground" the body to strengthen our connection of the lower dan tien and balance the flow of energy between the body and the head. Our frenetic culture often directs our energy upward into the head, leading to an unbalanced autonomic nervous system with excessive energy in the head, or upper dan tien. This shift of energy upward is further increased by illness, trauma, fear, stress, or grief.[8]

I learned about the ancient practice of toe tapping from Dr. Ann Marie Chiasson during my fellowship at the Andrew Weil Center for Integrative Medicine at University of Arizona. Dr. Chiasson has written about this in her book *Energy Healing: The Essentials of Self-Care*.[9] Toe tapping grounds the energy in the body by opening energy flow to the legs and hips and balancing the energy flow between the body and the head. From a TCM perspective, toe tapping energizes the spleen, liver, and stomach acupuncture channels, which enable overall vitality and energy. Toe tapping also stimulates return of venous blood flow to the heart and lymphatic flow from the legs.

Toe tapping can be done on a comfortable place on the floor. Or, if you have back problems, you can use a couch or bed. This activity is *not* for anyone who has had a recent knee or hip replacement or for anyone who is pregnant. If you fit into any of these categories, you can use a handheld vibrating massager on the feet and legs to stimulate flow to the lower body instead of doing this activity.

Lie flat on your back, hips loose and feet apart. Keeping your legs straight, swivel them from the hips like the windshield wipers on your car, in and out from your hips. Your heels will remain in one place on the floor. As your legs rotate in, tap your big toes together, then let your legs and feet swivel back out. Again, make sure to keep your legs straight, and swivel your legs from the hips, not from the ankles. Tap your toes together at as rapid a pace as you can, allowing momentum to make the exercise easier. You can relax and close your eyes. If you like, choose some music with a fast rhythm so you can tap to the beat. When you first begin this exercise, continue for five minutes; you can increase to as much as twenty minutes as you get used to it. Try it for at least a month.

Toe tapping can be used in the morning to increase energy to the lower body. You can also use it at night to shift excess energy from your head and settle your energy flow to relieve insomnia. The activity acts as an adaptogen—a therapy that brings the body into balance. The grounding effect from toe tapping is helpful for anxiety, as well as restless leg syndrome, neuropathic pain, and insomnia. When energy is low, this exercise can activate qi. When you are anxious, it can relax you.

So, here we have added several movement tools to integrate for relief from anxiety—moderate or vigorous aerobic activity, yoga, and toe tapping. Once you get the pathways to healing started, your body will begin to tell you what movement it needs. Most important, enjoy the movement!

From Phyllis

One of the reasons I find God's Word so helpful is that it is packed with stories about real people who had real problems. If you're familiar with the Bible, you already know there aren't many stories about saints found there, but there are plenty of stories about people who found themselves in dire situations that would cause anyone anxiety. Think about these: Noah facing the flood, Moses facing the Red Sea with an army approaching, King David fleeing his enemies, Queen Esther about to lose her entire family, and young unmarried Mary being told she would give birth to God's Son. These were anxiety-producing events that necessitated decisions.

Peter is one of my favorite Bible characters because he was a passionate, emotion-filled, flawed follower of Jesus. Peter had one of those chest-in-the-vise experiences that overwhelmed him with anxiety. It had been a stressful day—one of those roller-coaster days of emotion-packed highs and lows. Jesus and His disciples had learned of the death of John the Baptist, and they had withdrawn by boat to a remote area on the Sea of Galilee. But the people who lived in the nearby villages followed them on foot, and a large crowd gathered. Peter witnessed Jesus as He healed the sick and fed the multitude (see Matthew 14).

At the close of the day, Jesus instructed His disciples to get into the boat and cross to the other side of the lake while He went alone up into the mountains to pray. Night fell, the winds picked up, and the disciples found themselves in surging waves threatening to capsize their boat.

In the wee hours, during their struggle to stay afloat, they saw a ghostlike figure coming toward them on the water. This struck even more fear in them. Then, through the wind came a familiar voice as Jesus told them to take courage. But Peter was so riddled with fatigue and anxiety that he required proof it really was Jesus. He said, "Lord, if it's really you, tell me to come to you, walking on the water" (Matthew 14:28 NLT).

Jesus invited him to come, and Peter did a courageous thing in spite of his fear. He moved. He got out of the boat and started toward Jesus. Then he looked down at the crashing waves all around him and began to sink. But the end of that story is one that gives us hope. Jesus took Peter's hand, and they both climbed to safety back into the boat, and the waters calmed.

This was not Peter's last experience with anxiety and fear. Jesus did not insulate Peter from stressful situations, and He did not take those anxious feelings away from Peter once and for all. Instead, He offered Peter a way to deal with his anxious feelings: Jesus offered His presence. At times Peter doubted and denied, but he still experienced enough of the peace Jesus offered that he chose to follow Christ all the way to his death as a martyr. He experienced the presence of Christ in stressful times, and he offered us a word of hope: "Give all your worries and cares to God, for he cares about you" (1 Peter 5:7 NLT).

Perhaps you are experiencing some anxiety that is drowning you in despair. You may not be in a literal storm or in physical danger, but still, your anxious feelings come in surges and waves. At times, you feel they will overtake you, and you're in desperate need of something or Someone to bring you to safety. Just like He did with Peter, Jesus reaches out to you, offering you His hand, His presence, during your times of overwhelming anxiety. He may not always calm the water, but He can bring calm to you.

Be like Peter. Honestly express your fear and doubt, but take courage. Don't let your anxiety paralyze you. Also, understand that while God is there to help you, there are things He expects you to do. Get out of the boat you're in, and do your part to move toward wellness. Experience God's presence, and practice the things that you can do for yourself physically to help you deal with life's anxious moments.

Inhale

"Don't be afraid, for I am with you. Don't be discouraged, for I am your God. I will strengthen you and help you. I will hold you up with my victorious right hand."

(Isaiah 41:10 NLT)

"Every tomorrow has two handles. We can take hold of it with the handle of anxiety or the handle of faith."

(Henry Ward Beecher)

Exhale

Dear Father, I ask for an awareness of Your presence when I am anxious. I ask for courage to do my part to take steps toward experiencing Your peace. Help me realize that means taking care of my body and my mind. Amen.

Self-Care Steps to Calm

- Use enjoyable movement this week for calming. Take a brisk walk, preferably outdoors in nature, several times this week.

- If you practice yoga, try a yoga series outdoors, weather permitting. If you haven't practiced yoga, find an on-line video series and benefit from the focus on breathing.

- Try toe tapping in the morning or evening and see how this makes you feel, as you are activating your acupuncture meridians. Balance your body's energy in another step to calm.

Step Three

Foods to Decrease Anxiety

"Nutrition is the only remedy that can bring full
recovery and can be used with any treatment.
Remember, food is our best medicine."

Bernard Jensen

From Dr. Jan

Whether or not medication is needed for an individual's
anxiety, good nutrition is key in maintaining healthy
brain function and reducing anxiety. In general, the
Standard American Diet (SAD) is calorie dense but
nutrient poor. The SAD is high in refined sugar, refined
flour, red meat, processed meat, and other highly
processed foods.[1] Most of the adult US population do not
eat the recommended amount of vegetables daily.[2] The
US Department of Agriculture estimates that eighty to
ninety percent of the US population do not eat the
recommended two servings of seafood weekly.[3] Less
than thirty percent eat three or more vegetable servings
daily. High-carbohydrate and high-fat diets can lead to
obesity as well as anxiety.[4]

Nutritional deficiencies in the SAD are common, and
unless these are corrected, mental health can suffer.

When we discussed stress eating, we reviewed how high glycemic-index foods with refined sugar and high-fructose corn syrup like cookies, candy, and sugary drinks can give us a quick feel-good response, but then our blood sugar drops quickly, and sugar cravings return.

So, what should we be eating to counteract anxiety?

Dark leafy greens. Yes, you've seen these before in the Stress section! These include spinach, kale, parsley, broccoli, broccoli sprouts, Swiss chard, collard greens, Romaine lettuce, and arugula. These foods are high in antioxidants to protect us from oxidative stress and contain nutrients to support optimal brain function.[5] Vitamin E, vitamin C, vitamin E, beta-carotene, and folate are found in all of these greens as well. And research supports that dark, leafy greens give us protection against cognitive decline.[6]

In addition, dark leafy greens provide magnesium, a mineral that is crucial for many biochemical reactions in the body—something that is typically deficient in the SAD.[7] Magnesium helps to regulate neurotransmitters and is needed for muscle relaxation.

Foods containing omega-3 fatty acids. These are considered essential fatty acids, since we do not make them in the body but rely on dietary intake. Some studies have shown that regular consumption of these polyunsaturated fatty acids is helpful for mood disorders.[8] They are also heart healthy. The major omega-3 fatty acids are alpha-linoleic acid (ALA), eicosapentaenoic acid (EPA), and docosahexaenoic acid (DHA). The SAD diet contains insufficient omega-3s but many more omega-6 fatty acids, which are found in corn oil, vegetable oil, and many processed foods.

The main source of EPA and DHA are cold-water fish with these healthy fatty oils: wild salmon, cod, mackerel, sardines, tuna, halibut, and anchovies. Dairy products, eggs, meat, and poultry contain some omega-3s; grass-feeding increases the omega-3 content of these. Omega-3 supplements may also be used. Be sure and check with your health-care professional before starting a supplement.

For vegetarians or those who cannot eat fish, plant sources of omega 3s are found in flaxseed oil, walnut oil, canola oil, and wheat-germ oil. These contain ALA, which is a precursor to EPA and DHA. Walnuts and seeds such as chia seeds and flaxseeds are also good sources, but the flaxseed must be ground prior to eating to have good absorption of the omega-3s. These can be sprinkled on soups or salads or added to smoothies.

Purslane is another excellent plant source. It is easy to grow, even in pots, and can be added as a garnish to any dish. Spirulina has also been used as a source of omega-3s in vegetarians, but currently there is some concern about contamination with a neurotoxin in areas where algae blooms occur, and some experts no longer recommend it.[9]

Walnuts. Studies have correlated the intake of these nuts with improved mood.[10] In addition to being a source for ALA omega-3s, walnuts are a good source of magnesium and antioxidants. And they contain nutrients that protect cognitive brain function, such as vitamin E, melatonin, polyphenols, folate, and copper, as well as magnesium.

Herbs and spices. Herbs and plant spices such as rosemary, thyme, basil, clove, and cinnamon are powerful antioxidants. Add some, fresh or dried, to your recipes.

Turmeric is a powerful anti-inflammatory and has a neuroprotective effect on the brain.[11] Turmeric contains the active compound curcumin, which boosts the conversion of ALA into DHA. Curcumin has been shown in animal studies to decrease effects of anxiety.[12] Turmeric is better absorbed with piperine, a compound in black pepper, so use the two together.

Ginger is a root vegetable in the same family as turmeric. It is also a powerful anti-inflammatory and antioxidant and is useful for relieving nausea. It has also been shown to increase levels of serotonin, a calming neurotransmitter.[13]

Dark chocolate. Yes! Dark chocolate with at least 70 percent cocoa is good for you and can make you feel better quickly. Cocoa is rich in flavonoids, antioxidants, and polyphenols that have been shown to reduce stress and support heart health.[14] Most people are used to eating chocolate with a lot of refined sugar and poor-quality dairy ingredients. This type of chocolate can increase anxiety due to the stress-eating cycle we discussed. However, a one-ounce serving of high-quality dark chocolate is restorative.

Teas. Lemon balm (*Melissa officinalis*) is a lovely herb that is easy to grow in the garden or in a pot. It is in the mint family, and the leaves have a strong lemon scent. Whether in a tea or in herb or essential-oil form, it has a calming effect.

Green tea is made from the fresh tea leaves of *Camellia sinensis*. This form of tea contains beneficial catechins, flavonoids and theanine; the theanine has a calming effect. Green tea contains caffeine, but less than black tea.

Chamomile, as discussed in the section on Stress, also has a calming and even hypnotic effect.

Try all of these teas to see which works best for you.

Water. It is important to stay well hydrated. Dehydration makes us irritable and more anxious. You can judge how hydrated you are from the color of your urine. You should aim for it to be light yellow or almost colorless. Dark-yellow urine usually means you are volume depleted. Check with your health-care professional about any changes in your hydration or diet in case you have special considerations, especially if you have heart or kidney disease.

These are some highlights of foods that can relieve anxiety. And an overall healthy eating style is most supportive of that goal. Two excellent eating programs are the Mediterranean Diet and Dr. Weil's Anti-Inflammatory Diet.[15] Both of these eating plans have been associated with decreased chronic inflammation that leads to so many diseases. They both emphasize vegetables and fruits, which have been shown to be associated with lower rates of stress and better moods. We will discuss these diets more in the next section.

Healthy eating is really a lifestyle rather than a diet. It's about taking steps to improve your health, decrease your risk of chronic disease, and improve your sense of well-being.

If you are not ready to make drastic changes, you can take some small steps by eating more plants, for instance. We really are made up of what we put in our bodies, and our eating habits eventually catch up to us. Part of self-care is choosing to take care of yourself with healthy food choices.

From Phyllis

I recall the late afternoon when a friend and colleague, called obviously upset. She seemed to be laughing and crying at the same time. Her two little boys had wanted to be helpers and had asked to wash her car on that Saturday afternoon. Although they were only seven and four, she allowed them to wash the car because the weather was so hot, and she thought the boys would have fun with the water hose. So, she got out the soap and the buckets and handed them the hose.

Hours later, after the boys had finished and cleaned up, the family left for pizza at their favorite spot downtown. My friend's husband cranked the car, and it sputtered and buckled. They barely made it out of the driveway before the car stalled completely. Her husband got out and lifted the hood, trying to assess the problem. The youngest boy said to his mother, "It's not out of gas.

We filled the gas tank up this afternoon when we washed the car."

Gasp.

Do you know what happens when someone fills your gas tank with a water hose? Water and fuel don't mix. The fuel rises to the top, and as soon as the car has used up the fuel already in the line, there's nothing left but the water that has settled to the bottom. Engineers did not design car engines to run off water. Long story short, my friend's car had to be towed, and the fuel tank and fuel line had to be drained. Then the fuel filter had to be replaced. It was an expensive tank of something that didn't belong in a fuel tank.

Perhaps we can learn something about our bodies from this story. God was the Engineer who designed the human machine, and it seems perfectly logical that He would create the fuel that would make it run to its optimum. In Genesis we read, "The LORD God made all kinds of trees grow out of the ground—trees that were pleasing to the eye and good for food" (2:9 NIV).

Doctors and scientists have proven that the vegetables and fruits God provides are good for us, decreasing our odds of getting a dreaded disease. As Dr. Jan has written, some of these foods even help to decrease anxiety. And the foods that are good for you not only fuel your bodies, they can restore and help heal your bodies from the daily wear and tear and exposure to manmade toxins. On the other hand, science has shown that some of the additives and preservatives man has created cause many health issues for those who eat the Standard American Diet (SAD).

God's desire is for humans to be healthy and whole and to treat their bodies as His temple. He gives us what we need: "Then God said, 'Look! I have given you every seed-bearing plant throughout the earth and all the fruit trees for your food'" (Genesis 1:29 NLT). Think of those unhealthy items (I choose not to call them *food*) that you are eating as vandals and thieves. They are robbing you of your health, your healthy emotions, and perhaps even your longevity. God wants you well, but you must do your part. Choose healthy, life-giving foods on your path to wellness. You are God-made and worth it.

Inhale

"Eat food, not too much, mostly plants."

(Michael Pollan)

"Fruit trees of all kinds will grow on both banks of the river. Their leaves will not wither, nor will their fruit fail... Their fruit will serve for food and their leaves for healing."

(Ezekiel 47:12 NIV)

"Take care of your body. It's the only place you have to live."

(Jim Rohn)

Exhale

Dear Father, thank You for creating me and for providing for my needs. You, who created all there is, filled the earth with good things, for which I am thankful. Help me to be responsible by giving my body those things that are best for it. Amen.

Self-Care Steps to Calm

- For one week, keep a food diary to record what you eat. See how many vegetables and fruits you are eating. And then concentrate on adding some of the following to your diet.

- Add a dark, leafy vegetable to at least three meals in one week. Try spinach, kale, parsley, broccoli, broccoli sprouts, Swiss chard, collard greens, Romaine lettuce, or arugula.

- Concentrate on adding omega-3s to your diet by adding at least one serving of cold-water fish in one week. Choose from wild salmon, cod, mackerel, sardines, tuna, halibut, and anchovies. For vegetarians or those unable to eat fish, choose chia seeds, ground flaxseed, or purslane.

- Get adventurous and experiment with new herbs and spices as you cook. Remember, rosemary, thyme, basil, clove, and cinnamon are powerful antioxidants. Add some, fresh or dried, to your recipes. Try some seasonings like turmeric and ginger.

- Treat yourself to some walnuts and good dark chocolate.
- Make note of how this new eating pattern compares with your usual eating habits and how you feel eating in this new way.

Step Four

Turning to Spirit

"You don't have to control your thoughts; you just
have to stop letting them control you."
Dan Millman

From Dr. Jan

Due to life's challenges we will find ourselves anxious at
times. As we cope, the more we can quiet our minds and
turn inward to our spirit, the sooner we will find respite.
We talked about steps related to breathing, movement,
and nutrition that can decrease anxiety. These strategies
will set us up to turn to our spirit. Meditation and
mindfulness are self-care steps that can get us there.

You may be able to sit quietly and follow your breath
for five to twenty minutes, allowing yourself to just be
present and observe your thoughts. This allows you to
put things in better perspective. Some of us may find that
difficult, however, and guided meditations can be very
helpful. Even if our minds are racing, these can calm us
and help us contact our spirit. There are a number of
excellent apps and websites that are good sources for
guided meditations. See the Self-Care Resources section
for suggestions.

I have found essential oils to be helpful when I am meditating and seeking mindfulness. Essential oils are distilled from plants, or, in the case of citrus oils, they are extracted from the rind of the citrus fruit. Most of them smell wonderful, and they are increasingly used for other beneficial properties. (Note: essential oils are not FDA-approved to prevent, treat, or diagnose any medical condition.) I use them in an ultrasonic diffuser in the room where I meditate. I just add a few drops of essential oil and then water to the water receptacle in the diffuser, and the ultrasonic vibrations send the diluted essential oil out into the air.

Even if you don't have a diffuser, you can put a couple of drops of essential oil on a cotton ball as a passive diffuser. And if you don't have an essential oil, since citrus oils come from the rind, you can take a piece of the zest—the outermost part of the rind—and twist it to get the citrus-oil aroma.

Studies have shown that essential oils can alleviate anxiety due to a variety of causes. In a recent review, the some of the oils used were lavender, bitter orange (*Citrus aurantium*), bergamot, sweet orange (*Citrus sinensis*), rose, and Roman chamomile.[1] Lavender had the most benefit in that review, and many people find it helpful for calming.

I have found there is a lot of personal preference in essential oils. I like to use frankincense, an essential oil that has been used in worship and meditation since ancient times, and palo santo (with attention to using the *Bursera graveolens* species, which is not endangered) for meditation. Be sure and breathe through your nose to get the best benefit.

How do essential oils work to affect our minds? Smell is actually a chemical reaction. Molecules from essential oil are detected by the cells in the lining of the nose. This is then detected by the smell (olfactory) nerve, which travels from the nasal passages directly to the limbic system area of the brain. This is the most primitive part of the brain that processes our emotions and motivation. Some research indicates that as the molecules from these aromas reach our brains, they cause the release of serotonin and dopamine, neurotransmitters for calming and pleasure.[2] However they work, the effect can be very helpful as we turn to our spirits and calm our minds.

We were making Integrative Medicine rounds recently in the hospital and saw a patient who was getting ready to have her wound dressing changed at bedside. This had previously been done in the operating room under anesthesia, but her wound was small enough now that there was more risk than benefit in taking her to the operating room. She was very anxious about this dressing change, admitting that she was very afraid of the pain that would occur. We gave her a nasal inhaler with lavender and directed her to guided-imagery meditations that our hospital makes available. There was a meditation specifically for anxiety. She immediately tuned in. When we returned the next day, she told us that the meditation helped her tremendously, and she made it through the dressing change just fine. She was very grateful and felt this helped her more than medication could.

The mind is indeed very powerful. We just have to remember to use the tools that help us turn to our spirit.

From Phyllis

Ponder this: We are not human beings having a spiritual experience. We are spiritual beings having a human experience. That saying has been attributed to both French Christian philosopher Pierre Teilhard de Chardin and Wayne Dyer, a motivational speaker and author in the areas of self-help and spiritual development. Regardless of who first said it, the thought speaks to the notion that we are more than the physical. And both these men were interested in the idea of our souls—our total beings.

Can you imagine not existing? Just simply not being? Impossible. We can't imagine it. We were created as total beings with human bodies that exist while we're on this planet and spirits that are eternal. There are times we might wish we were someplace else or that our circumstances were different, but we still cannot wrap our heads around the idea of just not being.

The great Protestant theologian and philosopher of the twentieth century, Paul Tillich, wrote about nonbeing, fear, anxiety, and courage in his book *The Courage to Be*. Tillich spoke to the issue of anxiety and the fears we humans face. He concluded that our anxieties stem from our fears about death, emptiness and meaninglessness, and guilt.[3] It takes courage to live with these anxieties.

Often, when we think of courage, we think of some heroically brave act that would put us in the face of danger. Tillich does not look at courage as singular acts of bravery, but he sees real courage as an attitude, a disposition toward life.

If we are truly honest, there is much about life, existence, and the future that we do not and will never completely understand. Our everyday walking-around lives are riddled with many unknowns and a certain amount of risk. Even faith is a bit of a risky business. Faith is admitting that we don't have all the answers and we are dependent on someone or something outside ourselves. If we were absolutely certain of everything, we would have no need of faith.

Most of us do not have the mind and experience of Tillich or Chardin that will make us wise philosophers. And most of us will never risk like the Desert Fathers of the third century who left everything and everyone behind and moved to the desert to live a life of solitude and contemplation of spiritual matters. We may long for solitude and that kind of simplicity, but few of us will ever experience it. But perhaps Tillich, Chardin, and the Desert Fathers have something to teach us about the courage to live our lives and to move away from anxiety and toward wholeness and wellness.

God knows about our anxieties and that our bodies and spirits need rest. Jesus recognized this need in His disciples: "Then, because so many people were coming and going that they did not even have a chance to eat, he said to them, 'Come with me by yourselves to a quiet place and get some rest'" (Mark 6:31 NIV). Jesus knew what lay ahead for all of them, and He knew they needed rest and soul care.

Your heavenly Father knows your circumstances, and He knows what is ahead for you. He extends to you this same invitation to spend time with Him in a quiet place for some soul care. He doesn't desire that you be anxious or exhausted or overwhelmed. He wants you to give your mind and body a rest and time to recharge.

I choose to start every morning quietly reading Scripture, other inspirational readings, or poetry, and my hymnal is always near. God's Spirit speaks to my spirit during this time. And then I pray aloud to Him as though He were sitting next to me (because He is). Praying aloud keeps me centered and focused. Then I am ready for my day. This daily practice is part of my soul care, and it works for me.

Maybe it would help you to develop some practices that would serve as soul care for yourself—something that would relax your mind, calm your spirit, and build in you the courage to live with less anxiety. Perhaps taking a weekend or even an afternoon away from the busyness of your life and spending it in solitude might be a good place to start. If you find that arranging time away would cause you more stress, maybe you could take a long hike or a soak in your bathtub. Accept God's invitation to spend time with Him. After all, He made you a total being, body and spirit, and He knows how you live your best in this human experience.

Inhale

"Your calm mind is the ultimate weapon against your challenges."

(Bryant McGill)

"When anxiety was great within me, your consolation brought me joy."

(Psalm 94:19 NIV)

"Anxiety does not empty tomorrow of its sorrows, but only empties today of its strength."

(Charles Spurgeon)

Exhale

Pray: O God, thank You for the invitation to rest my body and calm my spirit. Help me find the balance and the courage to make time for the care of my soul. Amen.

Self-Care Steps to Calm

- Read about the benefits of using essential oils, and how to use them safely.
- Follow your breathing and diffuse an essential oil of your choice. If you don't have a diffuser, just use a cotton ball. For calming, lavender, orange, tangerine, blue tansy, or a combination of these can be beneficial.

- Listen to a guided meditation or guided imagery and see if this is helpful for your mindfulness. See Self-Care Resources for some suggestions.

- Treat yourself to an afternoon or evening escape. Take an hour for a relaxing hot bath. Lock the door and turn on relaxing music. Try to imagine peaceful scenes as you soak and breathe deeply giving care to yourself.

Step Five

Putting Self-Care Steps to Calm into Practice

"The greater the level of calmness of our mind, the
greater our peace of mind, the greater our ability
to enjoy a happy and joyful life."

Dalai Lama

From Dr. Jan

We have reviewed several powerful tools to control
anxiety. Start with intentional breathing. Take some time
in the morning, as you mentally and spiritually prepare
yourself to meet the day, to do your Coherent Breathing
or the 4-7-8 breath. See which works best for you. In the
evening, as you unwind, practice one of these again. As
you encounter stress or anxiety during the day, use the 4-
7-8 breath before you react. As you continue these
intentional breathing practices, you will find that you
consistently breath more deeply, slowly, and regularly
during the day as well.

Movement is a very powerful tool for counteracting
anxiety, and you can choose what is most enjoyable for
you. Moderate to vigorous activity can be very helpful in
getting your mind off worries. If you can choose an
outdoor activity, that may be even more beneficial for the

access to green spaces. Brisk walking, cycling, outdoor circuit training, jogging, and running are all excellent choices. You will need to check with your physician prior to starting any new physical activity. If you are not used to aerobic activity, start slow, go short distances, and build up to higher speeds and longer distances.

If aerobic activity is not for you, yoga is also a great choice, and there is evidence that it also shifts you into the relaxation response. If you would like to give it a try, there are many choices of on-line video series that can help you get started. Modifications in the movements may be needed when starting a yoga practice, so choose an instructor who discusses modifications during the session.

Think of toe tapping as an additional movement you can use as a movement meditation. Try it in the morning and in the evening, and see what works best for you. Begin with five minutes and work up to fifteen or twenty, as you like. If you are chronically anxious, try it for at least a month. Many people find this practice to be a powerful tool for self-care.

Finding time for movement is challenging until you incorporate it into your routine. Then you will wonder how you ever did without it.

It really is true that "You are what you eat." It's something to think about as we put food into our mouths. Do you want to be made of chips, crackers, cookies, alcohol, and processed foods? Or would you rather feed your body fuel that is high in antioxidants and have nutrients to support your brain and other organs in your body?

While a major change in diet may be difficult, you can take some self-care steps to healthier eating:

- Eat more vegetables (five servings daily) and fruits (two to three servings daily).
- "Eat the rainbow." See how many colors of vegetables and fruits you can eat.
- Include berries in the rainbow to increase your fiber intake.
- Choose a sweet potato instead of a white potato for more phytonutrients and vitamin A.
- See if you can eat thirty-five different vegetables and fruits in a week. Herbs and plant spices count!
- Check out the Environmental Working Group's Dirty Dozen, which indicates the foods that are most contaminated with pesticides.[1] For these plants, choose organic when you can to make sure they are chemical free.
- Use a variety of sources of protein, including beans and legumes (black beans, chickpeas, black-eyed peas, and lentils), dairy, and eggs.
- Include natural sources of omega-3s when you can, such as cold-water fish.
- Use other healthy fats such as olive oil, walnuts, pumpkin seeds, and avocado.
- Spice it up with healthy seasonings—turmeric, ginger, garlic, cinnamon, rosemary, thyme, and basil.
- Enjoy some dark chocolate with at least 70 percent cocoa.

- Coffee has some benefits as an antioxidant, but excess caffeine is associated with anxiety. More than one or two cups in the morning can increase anxiety for some people. Watch for this and notice how it affects you. It is usually a good idea to avoid drinking coffee throughout the day.

Taking some of these steps to change your eating patterns will involve a new grocery shopping list. You may find that you actually enjoy trying new things. Check out some delicious recipes at Dr. Weil's website.[2] Also check out the website of Liana Werner-Gray, who wrote the book *Anxiety Free with Food*.[3] After a few weeks of eating more vegetables, fruits, and anti-inflammatory foods, see if you have more energy, better concentration, and less anxiety.

In turning to spirit, we discussed using essential oils and guided meditations. If you haven't used essential oils before, you may want to give them a try. Because the molecules from essential oils go very quickly to the brain via the olfactory (smell) nerve and the limbic system, they can have a very rapid effect on mood and calming. For most people, lavender is a good oil to start with first. The citrus oils, especially orange and tangerine are also good for relaxation. Cedarwood is helpful for sleep. I have used a blend of lavender, orange, and cedarwood for sleep with good effect. Sandalwood and lemon balm (*Melissa officinalis*) are a bigger investment but they have lovely aromas and can reduce anxiety. Preferences in essential oils vary between person to person, so check out what works for you.

The best way to use essential oils, especially in the beginning, is aromatically—that is, by inhalation. An ultrasonic diffuser, as previously explained, is very easy and effective in diffusing aroma in a room. A nasal inhaler, also called an aroma stick, consists of a wick to which the oil of choice is applied and then inserted into the inhaler that can be held to the nose. Supplies for these can be ordered online (see Self-Care Resources). The aroma stick is especially useful since it is portable and can be pulled out at a moment of anxiety and used with a deep inhale to calm the mind. A cotton ball, as discussed previously, can also be used effectively as a passive diffuser.

A hot bath is also a way to destress. Another powerful way to use essential oils is to mix them into Epsom salts and put in the bath. Lavender is a good one to use for this. Start by putting a drop of lavender diluted in a teaspoon of carrier oil, such as vegetable oil, on the inside of your arm and observe to make sure you are not sensitive to lavender first. Then you can put four to five drops into two tablespoons of Epsom salts and drop that in a hot bath. Epsom salts are magnesium sulfate, which adds to the relaxation since magnesium relaxes the muscles.

There are a number of meditation apps that can be used for guided meditation. Some are for purchase and some are free. Insight Timer is one I use frequently.[4] One of my patients with chronic pain related that she was skeptical but found guided meditations for pain and for sleep very helpful. (She also told me that her cats loved the sleep meditation and kept pawing at her phone when it was on!) Among the numerous other meditation apps available, meditations can range from one minute to thirty minutes and longer. See options in the Self-Care Resources section; you can explore and find one you like best.

Prayer can also be very valuable in managing anxiety. Dr. Larry Dossey, a distinguished physician and influential advocate for the role of spirituality in health care, calls prayer an attitude of the heart. His book *Healing Words: The Power of Prayer and the Practice of Medicine* cites actual scientific experiments that have documented the healing power of prayer for spiritual people, which was not limited to certain religions.[5]

In my own life, I have found the guidance in Philippians to be true: "Do not be anxious about anything, but in every situation, by prayer and petition, with thanksgiving, present your requests to God. And the peace of God, which transcends all understanding, will guard your hearts and your minds in Christ Jesus" (Philippians 4:6–7 NIV). This does not mean my prayers have always been answered in the way I wanted; in fact, they have not. But the unloading of the burden of worries and problems to God can result in a peaceful soul.

Breathwork, movement, nutrition, essential oils, guided meditation, and prayer are powerful strategies you can use for self-care steps to calm. Using each of these with mindfulness will benefit your health.

From Phyllis

When we sense things are out of control or beyond our control, we experience anxiety. So many of our life experiences are beyond our ability to regulate, but how we give care to ourselves is. Dr. Jan has given careful instruction about some very practical things you can do to deal with your anxiety.

Some of the most anxious hours I've spent in the last few years have been in the doctors' offices awaiting a report, at home awaiting lab results, and in the cancer treatment center where my husband received chemotherapy and radiation. Some of those treatment days were fourteen hours of hand-wringing time, praying he would tolerate the medicines and not become violently ill. And then I'd have to take him home, where the next couple of days were critical and I alone was giving care. The fact that we were forty-five minutes from the medical center added to my anxiety.

And then there were the hours in the family waiting area of the hospital when he was in surgery. Aside from having a strong support system and my praying in those moments, I found that the essential oil clary sage was helpful to me. I dropped a few drops on a piece of felt and put it in my diffuser necklace. All through those times, I would periodically lift the locket and inhale the oil. I found it calming during very anxious hours.

Another helpful way of dealing with my anxiety was working at positive self-talk. Remember, the person who speaks to you the most is yourself, and those words you say to yourself really matter. Those words shape thought, which will become disposition and behavior. My positive way of speaking to myself not only shaped my thoughts but the way I spoke to my husband. You might consider filling your thoughts with positive, life-giving words.

You've probably noted already in this book that Dr. Jan and I appreciate good quotes. Use some of the quotes we have chosen, or do a quick internet search for quotes on dealing with anxiety. Choose a few of your favorites that speak to your spirit. Record them. You might put them on sticky notes and place them where they are reminders throughout the day.

If that doesn't work for you, choose one or two and memorize them, and when you sense that pang of anxiety, repeat that quote to yourself. When your own self-talk isn't helpful, allow someone else's encouraging, helpful words to shape your thoughts.

Of course, prayer is by far the most powerful resource we have. Think about it: the Creator of the universe, the Author of life, invites you to speak with Him. That is almost more than we can comprehend.

I am blessed with family and friends who also believe in the power of praying. When Bill was diagnosed with cancer, I mobilized a group of them to pray for him. I sent weekly Sunday-afternoon emails to that group of over fifty people who literally lived from coast to coast. My emails included a report on Bill, our prayer needs for the upcoming week, and an encouraging word of how we were experiencing God's presence and the answers to their prayers. Their responses and just knowing so many were praying for us calmed my anxiety and built a bond among us all. They prayed us through chemotherapy, surgery, radiation, and recovery. Now, three years later, I still communicate regularly with this praying group of family and friends.

You and I will always live in the shadow of cancer or whatever other challenges surround us, but we also live in the shadow of the wings of the Almighty One who invites us to cast our burdens and anxieties on Him. Not only does God invite us to speak with Him, He speaks to us through the encouragement of others and through His written word. I find that reading the Scripture and copying verses that resonate with my soul are most helpful to me. Not only are they positive reminders about what God desires for me, but the promises I find there allay my fears and give me assurance. Take a few minutes to start your day like Jesus did in talking with your Father and listening to Him through reading His Word.

Inhale

"Our bodies are our gardens—our wills are our gardeners."

(William Shakespeare)

"For God has not given us a spirit of fear and timidity, but of power, love, and self-discipline."

(2 Timothy 1:7 NLT)

Exhale

Dear Father, when I am fearful and anxious and feel control is slipping away, remind me that You are in control. Help me not to see my world through a lens of fear, and help me not to see self-care as being selfish. Amen.

Self-Care Steps to Calm

- Remember, breathe deeply and slowly.
- Your body was designed to move, so move. Stretch. Walk. Practice yoga. Enjoy tapping your toes, and make somebody laugh while you do.
- Avoid foods that feed your anxiety. Choose the foods that will give you the best health and most energy.
- Take time for self-care. If you can't take a weekend trip, escape for an hour for a soak in your tub.
- Let your self-talk be positive and encouraging and move you from fear to a sense of calm.
- Make an aroma stick (nasal inhaler) using your favorite essential oil for calming. You might start with lavender or clary sage. Order nasal inhalers online from wherever you would like to get your essential oil supplies (see Self-Care Resources). Put several drops of oil on the wick, then place the wick in the nasal inhaler. Click the bottom cap in place and screw on the top cap that covers the inhaler. Now you can keep it handy in your pocket or purse for use any time. It will last for several weeks.

Part Three

Self–Care for Depression

Step One

Depression

"I am now the most miserable man living. If what
I feel were equally distributed to the whole human
family, there would not be one cheerful face on the
earth. Whether I shall ever be better I cannot tell; I
awfully forebode I shall not. To remain as I am is
impossible; I must die or be better, it appears
to me."

Abraham Lincoln, age thirty-two

From Jan

The World Health Organization has rated depression as
the largest contributor to disability in the world.[1] Depression is common, affecting at least ten percent of US
adults, and up to twenty percent in some settings. It may
also affect five percent of teenagers.[2] While we all have
sadness or bad moods for short periods of time, depression is a medical condition that needs attention, to
address the biochemical changes in the brain that occur
with this disease.

The medical definition of *depression* includes five or
more symptoms present within a two-week period, of
which one of the symptoms is either a depressed mood

or loss of ability to experience pleasure/loss of interest. The other symptoms are change in appetite or weight (loss or gain), difficulties with sleep (too little or too much), agitation or slowing of movement, fatigue, inability to think or concentrate, feelings of worthlessness or guilt, or thoughts of suicide.[3]

Abraham Lincoln's quote, cited at the start of this section, from a letter he wrote to a friend, is a telling description of the despair and hopelessness that a depressed person can feel. Having been there myself, I can attest that depression feels like being at the bottom of a deep, dark pit with no foreseeable way of getting out.

Feelings and symptoms such as these warrant a medical evaluation, because there are diseases and nutrient deficiencies associated with depression that should be investigated. Traditional medical therapies for depression include newer antidepressants and psychotherapy. Some patients respond to antidepressant medications, but many do not. And these medications can have many side effects such as constipation, diarrhea, nausea, headache, dizziness, insomnia, and loss of libido. In some studies, psychotherapy has been judged to be as effective as antidepressants and has fewer side effects and lower relapse rates. Mental-health professionals are using an increasing number of therapies for treatment-resistant depression.

In any case, if you are depressed, treatment of your depression should be discussed with your physician. For a major depression, self-care strategies alone are usually not enough. There are actual biochemical changes in the brain, and antidepressant medication can be tremendously helpful. Whatever strategy is decided on, there are self-care strategies that can be integrated with medication and other traditional therapies.

What can intentional breathing offer here? Depression has been described as a low parasympathetic state, meaning that activation of the parasympathetic nervous system, or the relaxation response, can be of benefit. As we reviewed in Stress Step One, the vagus nerve helps to activate your parasympathetic nervous system.

Intentional breathing at a slower, deeper, more regular rate, can stimulate the vagus nerve and activate our relaxation response. It assists in developing mindfulness, that state of being in the present and in the moment and without worry about the past or the future. Ruminations—repeated negative thoughts about things that have happened and worries about what will happen—give way to calming as we follow the breath with mindfulness.

Brown and Gerbarg's book *The Healing Power of Breath* describes the sequence of Coherent Breathing, Resistance Breathing, and Breath Moving as the Total Breath.[4] Coherent Breathing is useful for activating the parasympathetic nervous system. This is the technique of slowing the breathing rate to five to six breaths per minute. The effect of this can be enhanced by Resistance Breathing, described by Brown and Gerbarg and others. Creating resistance during the breath increases the stimulation of the parasympathetic system. You may have learned Resistance Breathing in yoga, when it is often described as *ujjayi* breathing. It is also called the Ocean Breath, because the sound that is made is similar to the ocean sound heard in a seashell. To make this sound, make an *ahhh* sound when exhaling with your mouth open, then close your mouth to make the sound in the back of your throat on exhale. It is like making a sigh with the muscles tightened at the back of the throat.

In yoga, this breath helps to warm the body. It also enhances activation of the relaxation response. As you begin this practice, use it for a few minutes of your Coherent Breathing, and you can build up to a longer time.

The resistance breath leads to Breath Moving.[5] This is a practice to engage the mind in moving awareness to different parts of the body, which can increase energy flow and open energy centers in the body. The exercise has ancient roots in China and was further developed by Russian Christian Orthodox Hesychast monks in the eleventh century to prepare themselves for meditation and prayer.

Breath Moving can be calming as well as activating. You may find it most useful in the mornings if it is activating for you. Begin your Coherent Breathing, breathing in and out through the nose, and relaxing your body. For Circuit 1, as you inhale, picture your breath moving to the top of your head. As you exhale, picture your breath travelling to the base of your spine. Repeat this for ten cycles.

For Breath Moving Circuit 2, as you inhale, picture your breath moving to the top of your head. As you exhale, picture your breath travelling down your body and out through the bottom of your feet. Repeat this for ten cycles. Then repeat Circuit 1.

Vibration using the voice is another way to stimulate the vagus nerve and the relaxation response.[6] Vocalizing and humming the *m* sound and lower tone sounds are more effective than other sounds in causing vibration in the rest of the body. This is the rationale for the use of the classic *om* sound for meditation. There are similar sounds that can be used such as *shalom* (Hebrew), *salaam* (Arabic), and the word *amen*, which has both the *ahh* and *m* sounds. Use one of these words as you exhale in slow breathing. The effect of vibration on the vagus nerve travels to different parts of the brain, including those involved in processing emotions. Therefore, using one of these sounds in three exhalations at the beginning of your breathing practice can be beneficial.

Also, vocalizing with a group, whether live or with a recording, can also be therapeutic. If you are depressed, you may not always feel like singing. But if you can, use your voice with a group and see if your mood benefits.

From Phyllis

Suffering and sadness seem to be a part of the human experience. Not one of us is immune—not the wisest, kindest, richest, meanest, most powerful or powerless, and not even the most saintly folks. For those of us who have experienced the darkness of depression or who love someone who has, we know that depression is real.

The Bible is rich with stories about real people who suffered from depression. I find the prophet Elijah a most interesting person who survived one drama after another. Elijah lived in the northern kingdom of Israel in the eighth century BC and was chosen by God to deliver some straight-up news to the leaders of the day—namely the wicked King Ahab who had led the people away from God and to the worship of Baal, a false god. Elijah delivered the bad news that a drought was coming, and then he followed God's instruction to return to the desert, where God provided for his need of food and water: "The ravens brought him bread and meat each morning and evening, and he drank from the brook" (1 Kings 17:6 NLT). Because of the drought, the brook dried up. But God still provided. He told Elijah to go into a certain village where he would find a widow who would give him food and shelter.

During the of course his life, Elijah witnessed many miracles. Through his prayer, a young boy who had died came back to life. Then, when he asked King Ahab to allow the prophets of Baal to set up a demonstration on Mount Carmel to prove once and for all who the true God was, Elijah saw God miraculously reveal himself to His people through fire.

There is a good reason that very few people name their daughters Jezebel, for she was the evil and manipulative wife of King Ahab and queen of the land who was behind Ahab's actions. After the miracle on Mount Carmel, she sent Elijah the message that she would see to it that he be killed the very next day. Even with all that he had seen God do, Elijah fled in fear. He went a day's journey into the wilderness alone where, "He sat down under a solitary broom tree and prayed that he might die. 'I have had enough, LORD,' he said. 'Take my life, for I am no better than my ancestors who have already died'" (1 Kings 19:4 NLT). But the good news is this: even when Elijah was at the point of totally giving up, God did not give up on him.

I invite you to take a few minutes and read the story of Elijah in 1 Kings 17 through 19. This story gives me hope—real hope. As I wrote earlier, the Bible is not filled with stories about perfect saints, but instead with stories of real people who experience the same emotions we do. Elijah was a great man of God, and yet he was afraid. He was completely done and felt he could take no more. He suffered such depression that he even prayed to die.

If one who had seen miracles could still have the same emotions and struggles we do, then we have hope. Likely, none of us will wake every morning with fresh bread and water supplied by unseen hands, or see someone raised from the dead, or see God rain down fire on a water-soaked altar, or be chased into the wilderness by someone who is out to kill us, but we still experience fear and the depths of depression. At times we feel we are in a barren wilderness as we sit under our own broom tree.

So what can we learn from the story of Elijah?

- When Elijah had needs, God provided.
- When Elijah needed help, God provided others to help him.

- When Elijah was afraid, he prayed.
- When Elijah did not know if God would do what He said, he trusted.
- When Elijah was so depressed, he was honest with God and admitted it.
- When Elijah looked at the world through his own narrow lens and perspective, God helped him see things differently.
- When Elijah's fear and depression isolated him, God was still near.
- And most important, when Elijah was ready to give up, God never gave up on him.

God provides for us too. He brings hope. Although there are some important life lessons we can learn from Elijah, you should never, ever feel guilty if your depression is not taken away through prayer. You should never feel that God isn't listening because your faith is lacking. I still encourage you to pray and be honest with God about your feelings.

God, being the gracious, caring One that He is, gives us more than prayer to help us. Sometimes, He provides help through medicine, and often, He gives us practices that we can use to help ourselves. And remember: when you feel like giving up, God will never leave you alone, and He will never give up on you.

Inhale

"Moving the breath relaxes and refreshes, like an internal massage and shower."

(Dr. Richard P. Brown)

"So God has given both his promise and his oath. These two things are unchangeable because it is impossible for God to lie. Therefore, we who have fled to him for refuge can have great confidence as we hold to the hope that lies before us. This hope is a strong and trustworthy anchor for our souls. It leads us through the curtain into God's inner sanctuary."

(Hebrews 6:18–19 NLT)

"O LORD, you are my lamp. The LORD lights up my darkness."

(2 Samuel 22:29 NLT)

Exhale

Pray: Father, my fears are so real, and often I feel I'm wandering around in the dark, searching for a safe way out into the light. I ask You to be my strength and my light. I ask You, Lord, to return my hope. Amen.

Self-Care Steps to Hope

- In your meditation time, use Brown and Gerbarg's Total Breath, with Coherent Breathing, Resistance Breathing, and Breath Moving, for fifteen minutes.

Measure your heart rate before you start the Total Breath. Follow your breath during this time and let distracting thoughts go. Measure your heart rate afterward, and see if there is any difference.

- At another time during the day, sing a song, preferably one in low tones and with *m*'s and "amens" for the best vibrations. Even better, sing along with someone, even if it's online or virtual. Do you feel more light-hearted after singing?

Step Two

How Can I Move When I'm Depressed?

"Mental pain is less dramatic than physical pain,
but it is more common and also more hard to bear.
The frequent attempt to conceal mental pain
increases the burden: it is easier to say 'My tooth is
aching' than to say 'My heart is broken.'"

C. S. Lewis

From Dr. Jan

There is a great deal of evidence to show that physical activity can lessen the burden of depression. Depression, sedentary behavior, and cardiovascular disease are an important associated triad.[1] Both lack of activity and symptoms of depression have been shown to increase the risk of death from cardiovascular disease, but those with both risk factors have a higher risk of mortality. The protective effect of physical activity has been demonstrated across multiple ages and continents.[2]

There is no one type of activity that is best for everyone. Especially when depressed, it is helpful for the movement be enjoyable. Vigorous aerobic activity, such as running or swimming, is very helpful for relieving depression in some people. Moderate activity, such as a brisk walk or even gardening, can also be helpful. As we discussed in Step Two under Anxiety, current recommendations are for 150 minutes or more of moderate activity weekly or 75 minutes or more of vigorous activity, in addition to resistance training that strengthens muscles on two days a week.[3] The 150 minutes a week can be done in thirty-minute intervals five days a week, but those thirty minutes in a day do not have to be done at once. For instance, it can happen in two intervals of fifteen minutes each.

Depression increases with age, and physical activity can become less vigorous with age.[4] There is increased evidence that balance and strength training may be most beneficial in the older age group. Strength training, yoga, and tai chi have been shown to be beneficial to lessen symptoms of depression.[5] Strength training has the additional benefit of improving function and increasing bone density. Yoga and tai chi have can be successful in decreasing chronic back pain, and tai chi has been shown to decrease the incidence of falls, so these types of movement can be especially helpful in the older age group.[6]

In a recent study, yoga combined with Coherent Breathing was shown to significantly reduce symptoms of depression after a twelve-week program of sessions.[7] In addition, yoga has been shown to increase levels of gamma aminobutyric acid (GABA), a calming neurotransmitter, in the thalamus, a part of the brain influencing mood.[8] A deficit of this neurotransmitter is thought to contribute to mood disorders like depression.

The effect of increased GABA was sustained with at least one yoga session a week.

So, it's great to know that movement can relieve depression. But who feels like doing physical activity when they're depressed? Depression of the mind often extends to the body, with lethargy and disinterest as a result. Several strategies can help. Connect with a friend that you enjoy talking with. Take a walk with them just to talk, and make it a brisk walk if you can. In addition to the walk, you may find that talking to someone is therapeutic. Taking the first step to make the plan and do it is often the hardest step. Get a regular walk with a friend on your schedule to make it a habit.

Another opportunity is to volunteer to be the one to walk the family dog. Or, if you don't have a dog, see if you can walk your neighbor's dog. They may need the help. Or volunteer at an animal shelter. Caring for a pet can make you feel good because the dog will really appreciate it.

After you are used to walking, get other activities you like on the calendar. Try yoga, cycling, swimming, or weight training with a friend. Having an exercise buddy makes activity more fun and increases the chances that you will do it. Try a new activity for a lift. I recently discovered cardio drumming. It just takes a large exercise ball placed in a laundry basket, and a set of drumsticks. I found cardio drumming routines to music online, but I usually just make up my own routines to my music playlists. It is an enjoyable and different way to get moderate to vigorous activity. I also find that the drumming is a good way to relieve stress!

Finally, massage with moderate pressure has been shown to decrease depression and anxiety.[9] The effect on the body is the relaxation response: vagal tone increases, the heart rate goes down, and the level of our stress hormone, cortisol, decreases. Especially if you are increasing your activity level, a massage can be a welcome intervention.

From Phyllis

King Solomon is another interesting character from the Old Testament, and the author of the Song of Solomon, Ecclesiastes, and many of the Proverbs, known as Wisdom Literature. The son of King David and Bathsheba, Solomon was the third king of Israel. In his day, he was known as the wisest and the wealthiest king on earth. He was a builder. He built the temple in Jerusalem along with roads, trade, government buildings, and houses for his seven hundred wives and three hundred concubines. In the early days of his rule, he asked God for wisdom to be able to rule his people justly and honestly, but over time he was led away from God by his wives and concubines who did not worship Jehovah. His love for God waned, and so did his purpose for living.

Even with his wisdom and wealth, Solomon found himself in a dark place, where life had lost its meaning. He recognized the futility in pleasure and viewed his accomplishments as meaningless. Solomon said, "So I came to hate life because everything done here under the sun is so troubling. Everything is meaningless—like chasing the wind" (Ecclesiastes 2:17 NLT). Solomon had lost all hope and purpose, and he despaired.

I've had feelings and thoughts that resonate with King Solomon's. In the summer of 2018, after my husband was diagnosed with cancer for the second time, he immediately went into chemotherapy treatment in preparation for the removal of his kidney four months later. After the surgery, there were complications as his body felt the effects of the chemotherapy and worked to find its new homeostasis—a new state of balance and equilibrium.

For eighteen months, I was his caregiver as we basically hibernated to protect him, since his immune system had been compromised. There were the treatments, hospital stays, doctors' checkups, physical therapy, waiting for the next lab reports, and never-ending responsibilities at home. At times, I just wanted to curl up and pull the covers over my face. I felt fear and sadness, and the never-ending stress made me so tired and weary.

There were the nights when I would walk out on our deck and cry alone, looking into a black velvet sky and wondering if the morning would ever come again. And there were the low times when all seemed so futile, and hope seemed far away. But I knew that to be able to care for my husband as I wanted to, I needed to care for myself, and that included daily exercise.

I am a list maker. Even after years of retirement, I still maintain a day planner and calendar. Seeing those checkmarks at the end of the day gave me a sense of accomplishment. So, I started putting thirty minutes of daily exercise on my calendar just so I could feel I had done something. My sweet husband would sit in the sunshine on the deck and watch me as I walked the circular paths through the hills—paths we were accustomed to walking together. Since going to the gym was not an option, I also chose a thirty-minute Pilates routine that I did three times a week.

At first, the exercising was something else I had to do. But then I began to notice the benefits. I was sleeping better. The stretching and breathing and working my muscles helped me get rid of tension and the normal aches and pains of aging. After a short while, I actually found myself looking forward to the walking and the Pilates. I also chose to pray. On many of my walks, I talked to God out loud as though He was my walking companion. He was, you know.

Maybe you have (or have had) feelings similar to the loss of purpose and meaningless that Solomon experienced. Maybe you find yourself in a place where you have little control over the circumstances, and you feel hopeless and that you have no choice. Choosing to move, to exercise, is something you can control. As Dr. Jan advises, choose something that would be enjoyable to you, and choose a friend to join you. There are all kinds of positive benefits.

And trust God—not your feelings—and pray. Remember, it was King Solomon who also penned these words:

Trust in the LORD with all your heart;
>   do not depend on your own understanding.
Seek his will in all you do,
>   and he will show you which path to take. (Proverbs 3:5-6 NLT)

Inhale

"I pray that God, the source of hope, will fill you completely with joy and peace because you trust in him. Then you will overflow with confident hope through the power of the Holy Spirit."

(Romans 15:13 NLT)

"Do you not see how necessary a world of pains and troubles is to school an intelligence and make it a soul?"

(John Keats)

"A vigorous five-mile walk will do more good for an unhappy but otherwise healthy adult than all medicine and psychology in the world."

(Dr. Paul Dudley White)

Exhale

Pray: Father, there are times when I feel that I am practically paralyzed with dread, fear, and hopelessness.

Help me to trust You and not my feelings. Help me to make the choices that will move me from these feelings to a more hopeful place where I trust You completely. Amen.

Self-Care Steps to Hope

- Call a friend and set a time to take a walk with them.
- On a different day, choose an activity that you don't usually do, and try it this week. If you can, opt for something that gets your heart rate up and involves music.
- Find a good massage therapist who uses moderate pressure for an additional way to relax.
- End the week with a yoga class online or in a group to stretch and relax. Focus on your intentional breathing and *ujayyi* breath during your session.
- Make sure you talk to your doctor about your depression.

Step Three

Are You What You Eat?

"Tell me what you eat,
and I will tell you who you are."
Jean Anthelme Brillat-Savarin

From Jan

Brillat-Savarin was an eighteenth-century French lawyer and politician who is best known as an epicure and gastronome.[1] A food lover. While his claim to know who you are based on what you eat seems overreaching, it is absolutely true that what we eat predicts who we are.

What does this have to do with depression? There is a growing body of evidence that an unhealthy diet of processed foods, fried foods, refined grains, sweets, and refined sugar is associated with depression. And a healthy diet consisting of vegetables, fruit, fish, and lean meats is associated with a reduced risk of depression. While diet alone is not a primary treatment for depression, it is something you have control over, and it can be a helpful adjunct to psychotherapy and/or pharmaceuticals.

An increasing number of studies have shown an association with unhealthy food and increased risk of depression, as well as healthy eating with decreased risk of depression.[2] The explanation for this may be due to the higher antioxidant levels produced by a healthy diet that could decrease injury and stress to brain cells. Also, the protection of folate from vegetables and fruits can provide beneficial chemicals for brain function. Finally, fish consumption and the inclusion of omega-3 fatty acids can benefit the brain by preserving brain-cell membrane integrity and decreasing inflammation. Some studies suggest that consumption of fruit, vegetables and/or fish is especially protective against depressive symptoms.[3] There were some initial studies suggesting the benefit of omega-3 supplements for depression, but a recent randomized clinical trial showed that these supplements do not prevent depression.[4]

Let's discuss a couple of eating lifestyles in a little more detail. The Mediterranean Diet is so named because it reflects the food eaten by those in the countries bordering the Mediterranean Sea, including Greece and Italy, whose inhabitants were observed to have longevity and lower rates of cardiovascular disease and other chronic health conditions.[5] This nutrition style features complex carbohydrates such as whole grains and legumes, vegetables and fruits, fatty fish with omega-3 fatty acids such as salmon or tuna, healthy fats to include nuts and olive oil, and sweets such as dark chocolate and red wine in moderation. There are studies suggesting that the Mediterranean diet can improve mental health.[6] This eating style has been shown to contribute to the prevention of other brain diseases as well as depression.[7]

Dr. Weil's Anti-Inflammatory Diet is based largely on the same principles as the Mediterranean Diet, with some extras like green tea for its super antioxidant benefits.[8] As mentioned before, green tea comes from the *Camellia sinensis* plant, which is also the source of black tea. Black tea is fermented, however, and green tea is not. It is made from freshly harvested tea leaves that are heated and then dried. This preserves the valuable polyphenols and catechins in the tea leaves, which are powerful antioxidants thought to help in the prevention of heart disease and cancer.

Green tea can promote an "alert calm" due to the presence of some caffeine but also L-theanine, which gives a calming effect. This combination can also improve brain function and elevate mood. A few things to note: Trusted sources of green tea are important, to avoid those contaminated with pesticide exposure. Also, taking a supplement with a concentrated amount of catechins can result in high levels that may inflame the liver, but this would be rare from just ingesting the tea.

We have expounded on the benefits of dark chocolate elsewhere, but a high-quality dark chocolate with seventy percent cocoa is full of polyphenols and flavonoids that help protect the heart, benefit the metabolism, and improve mood and cognition. A study showed that eating dark chocolate regularly was associated with a seventy percent decrease in risk of depressive symptoms.[9] The same benefit was not seen with milk chocolate.

The Mediterranean Diet, Anti-Inflammatory Diet, and other healthy eating patterns all include fatty fish with omega-3 fatty acids. We noted this before but it bears repeating that omega-3 polyunsaturated fatty acids are essential in the diet, since the body cannot make its own. Two kinds of omega-3 fatty acids are found in fish—eicosapentaenoic acid (EPA) and docosahexaenoic acid (DHA). Sources include salmon, mackerel, herring, tuna, halibut, lake trout, anchovy, lake white fish, and sea bass. The American Heart Association recommends eating at least two servings of fish a week.[10] Fish that contain mercury, such as tuna, should be eaten less often—not more than twice a month.

For vegetarians or those who cannot eat fish, the omega-3 fatty acid alpha-linolenic acid (ALA) is found in plant sources such as ground flaxseed, flaxseed oil, chia seeds, walnuts, pumpkin seeds, purslane, soy foods, canola oil and algae oil. Not as many studies have been done with ALA as with EPA/DHA, but it is also thought to be beneficial.

In addition to supporting brain health, omega-3 fatty acids can reduce the risk of cardiovascular disease, lower triglyceride levels, raise high-density lipoprotein (HDL or "good" cholesterol), and lessen inflammation. So, including omega-3s in your diet is good for your health.

A deficiency of the B vitamins has also been associated with depression.[11] Folic acid is essential for healthy emotions and normal brain-cell function, and low levels of folate have been observed in depression.[12] It affects the production of neurotransmitters in the brain, which are critical in avoiding depression. Food sources of folic acid include dark leafy greens, chickpeas, beans, asparagus, avocado, and whole grains.

Vitamins B6 (pyridoxine) and B12 (cyanocobalamin) are also essential for normal brain function, and deficiencies of these have also been associated with depression.[13] Food sources of B6 include chickpeas, tuna, salmon, chicken breast, and fortified breakfast cereal. Vitamin B12 is found in lean animal products such as trout, salmon, and tuna, as well as milk. It is also found in fortified breakfast cereal. Vegans and the elderly are usually most at risk for B12 deficiency and may need a supplement. Check with your doctor about B-vitamin supplements if you cannot eat these food sources.

Low levels of vitamin D have also been associated with depressed mood.[14] The active form of vitamin D is created in the skin after sun exposure, and people at risk for vitamin D deficiency include the elderly who don't get outside much as well as those with melanin-rich skin. Those living at higher latitudes in the winter months can also become deficient in vitamin D. If you are in a risk group, check with your doctor about supplementing Vitamin D.

Vitamin D deficiency can contribute to seasonal affective disorder, a depressed mood that occurs during the winter when people have less sun exposure.[15] There are many factors at play in this disorder, including a change in the biological clock and a drop in serotonin and melatonin. Bright-light therapy during the season when this occurs can be helpful and should be done in conjunction with your doctor.

Deficiencies of certain micronutrients and minerals can also contribute. Low selenium levels have been associated with depression.[16] However, this is not a common problem in this country. Food sources of selenium include Brazil nuts, seafood, eggs, whole grains, and poultry. Selenium supplements can lead to toxicity, so it is best to get this mineral from food.

Chromium is also of interest in depression.[17] This mineral is an antioxidant and supports the action of insulin. A diet high in refined sugars, common in the Standard American Diet, increases the excretion of chromium and could result in deficiency. Chromium also supports the function of the "feel good" neurotransmitter in the brain: serotonin. This action may explain the improvement in mood seen in several studies when chromium was supplemented. And the metabolic effect on insulin may explain the decrease in carbohydrate cravings seen in some studies. Food sources of chromium include whole grains, eggs, grape juice, orange juice, beef, poultry, ham, and bananas. Brewer's yeast is also a good source and can be added to foods.

A recent study of young adults with symptoms of depression showed that a diet intervention of healthy eating for three weeks resulted in significantly fewer depressive symptoms compared to a control group without such an intervention that had no change in symptoms.[18] The healthy diet consisted of the Mediterranean-style diet with vegetables, fruits, whole-grain cereals, lean protein, unsweetened dairy, nuts and seeds, olive oil, and the spices turmeric and cinnamon. The non-intervention group continued to eat a diet high in refined carbohydrates, processed and fried foods, and sugary foods and beverages. Of note, reduction in processed foods contributed most to the reduction in depressed mood. Examples of processed foods included those that come in a package with multiple ingredients and foods with more than ten grams of sugar per one hundred grams, to include sodas, sweets, and fried takeaway foods. Even moderate compliance with the healthy diet was beneficial; strict compliance was not necessary for benefit. This means that even small to moderate changes can be beneficial for our moods.

An important aspect of healthy eating is minimizing processed foods with refined sugar. Too much sugar has been shown to decrease brain-derived neurotrophic factor (BDNF), a deficiency that has been associated with depression and anxiety.[19] BDNF is critical for healthy brain cells, memory, and brain plasticity—the ability of the brain to adapt to new learning. And, as we have reviewed previously, refined sugar can start the cravings that result in high and low blood-sugar cycles.

We are also learning more about the microbiome-gut-brain axis. The microbiome is comprised of the trillions of bacterial organisms in the gastrointestinal tract—more than ten times the number of human cells in the body. It functions to establish and maintain the intestinal lining, but we are learning that it can do much more. The makeup of the microbiome is affected by genetics, gender, and age, as well as diet.[20]

Studies in recent years have shown an association of the microbiome composition with many conditions, including stress and depression.[21] Certain bacterial species have been missing from the microbiome of people with depression.[22] In general, a diverse and stable microbiome is thought to be important for health and wellness. Research has shown that eating more than thirty types of plants a week is associated with a more diverse and stable microbiome.[23]

The role of probiotics—live beneficial bacteria taken orally as a supplement—has been studied as an intervention in depression.[24] Commonly used probiotics include some species of *Lactobacillus*, *Bifidobacterium*, and/or *Saccharomyces boulardii*. Some of these beneficial bacteria can also be found in fermented foods, such as yogurt with live cultures, kefir, kombucha, kimchi, and sauerkraut.

Studies are very preliminary, but some show that a probiotic supplement is associated with improved mood and cognition and decreased anxiety in patients with depression. As a mechanism, probiotics have been associated with an increase the expression of BDNF, which is reduced in patients with depression.[25] They have also been shown to increase production of GABA (gamma-aminobutyric acid), a calming neurotransmitter.[26] In addition, they may increase the production of serotonin, a neurotransmitter involved in regulating emotions and stress, by increasing the availability of a serotonin precursor, tryptophan, in the gut.[27] Serotonin is the target of the most commonly used antidepressants, selective serotonin reuptake inhibitors (SSRIs).

All of this information can be a bit overwhelming to read through, with its many scientific names and chemical interactions and acronyms. What's most important to take away is that, although the field of nutritional psychiatry is still emerging, it is evident that eating a diverse diet that follows the principles of the Mediterranean Diet or the Anti-Inflammatory Diet, with vegetables, fruits, nuts, healthy oils, fish, and lean meat, is not only good for our body but also for our brains and our mood. Conversely, diets high in processed foods and refined sugar are detrimental to mood as well as our overall health. Even moderate adherence to these principles can be of benefit.

From Phyllis

Depression can rob us of many things—sleep, energy, purpose, appetite, joy... It can also change our eating habits. So, I ask you a few questions: Are you eating mindlessly or with mindfulness? Are you eating because you're really hungry? Are you grabbing something because it's easy? Are you intentionally choosing something good for you?

For many years, I took the privilege of grocery shopping and the variety of foods available to me for granted. Although I did enjoy cooking, it was more of a chore and responsibility. An experience I had on a June morning in the highlands of Guatemala changed my attitude. Bill and I were leading a mission team of sixteen to spend a week working in an orphanage. Five precious Capuchin nuns, who had taken a vow of poverty, were taking care of all the needs of twenty-seven girls ages six to eighteen, and we were there to help.

The orphanage was located in the small, rural, and poverty-stricken village of Salcajá. The nuns had secured a small home where all thirty-two of them lived. I have many memories of these experiences, but none like the morning I spent in the kitchen with Sister Gabriela, affectionately known as Sister Gabby.

I had checked on all the activities and team members, and everything was running like a well-oiled machine, so I went to the kitchen to find Sister Gabby. Her pure voice singing her praises in beautiful Spanish greeted me before I opened the door to this kitchen, which was about the size of my walk-in clothes closet at home. She prepared three meals a day for thirty-two in a kitchen with a two-burner stove, three feet of work surface above the one cabinet, no sink or running water, and limited pots and pans.

When I went in, Sister Gabby had two large pots of boiling water on the stove, and she was chopping a cabbage the size of a basketball with a large knife like it was the most enjoyable thing she had ever done. That rusty knife was so old and primitive that I couldn't tell the sharp side from the dull side. But she was singing, and I could hear the happiness of her heart.

When I entered the kitchen, she pointed to the floor just inside the door. There was a large bag, the kind of netted bag our grocery-store onions come in. In the bag were four cabbages, a few onions, and maybe a dozen carrots the size of my forearm. I had never seen such large vegetables. In an excited voice, she said, *"Mira lo que Dios proporcionó."* Look what God has provided. *"Tendremos sopa para el almuerzo."* Now, we will have soup for lunch.

As I helped her scrape carrots with another dull knife, I learned that the sisters had asked God in their early-morning prayers for His provisions for the day, and God had provided through the gifts of a local farmer who showed up just in time. Sister Gabby's gratitude was written all over her face as she made a simple soup. I saw her joy and remembered that I often looked at food preparation as no more than something else I had to do.

After committing to better nutrition for health reasons, I now choose and prepare food with more intentionality—making wiser choices about fruits, vegetables, grains, and lean meats. But after my experience with Sister Gabby, I now enjoy the prep for cooking, as I have become mindful and grateful for different colors, flavors, and textures—the shiny smoothness of the aubergine eggplant, the orange of the carrot, the deep burgundies of fresh beets, the varieties of colors and shapes of squash, and the different shades of green in leafy vegetables. And just think how many varieties of apples are in the produce aisle. God provides such a variety of good things for us. You will always find a basket of fresh fruit on my counter because we like to eat it, but also because the fruits are just as beautiful as flowers to me.

I enjoy cooking. It's creative and is like therapy. There is instant gratification in the process. So I challenge you to be more intentional as you shop and prepare the foods you eat. Experiment with vegetables you've never tried, like a rutabaga or rhubarb. Try some new spices or a new recipe. Make shopping and preparing food a delightful, mindful experience. It can be fun. Then reap the rewards of your work as you eat.

God has given us what we need to fuel our bodies to run efficiently. He wants you to make choices that would keep you healthy. When you are mindful of His provisions for you, perhaps your grateful heart will be lifted just a bit like Sister Gabby's.

Inhale

"Whatever is good and perfect is a gift coming down to us from God our Father, who created all the lights in the heavens. He never changes or casts a shifting shadow."

(James 1:17 NLT)

"The spirit cannot endure the body when overfed, but, if underfed, the body cannot endure the spirit."

(St. Frances de Sales)

"Getting better from depression demands a lifelong commitment. I've made that commitment for my life's sake and for the sake of those who love me."

(Susan Polis Schutz)

Exhale

Pray: Dear Father, I marvel at all Your provisions when it comes to the foods that I eat, the varieties of foods available to me, and the abundance of it. I ask for Your help in making the wisest choices that would keep me healthy and productive. Make me mindful so that I am always able to express my gratitude to You. Amen.

Self-Care Steps to Hope

- How are you eating these days? Keep track of the servings of vegetables and fruit that you have daily. Aim for a least five servings of vegetables and two servings of fruit.
- If you can eat fish, include oily fish rich in omega-3 fatty acids in your meal twice a week.
- Try some green tea instead of coffee for your mid-morning break.
- Use nuts, including walnuts, a source of omega-3s and magnesium, as a healthy snack instead of processed food sources with refined sugar.
- As you prepare your food, be mindful of the look, smell, and feel of the vegetables and fruit. Thank God for the variety of foods and food sources He provides.

Step Four

The Poor in Spirit

"Blessed are the poor in spirit, for theirs is the
kingdom of heaven."

Matthew 5:3 NIV

Dr. Jan

Depression is a disease of mind, body, and spirit. The
mind is foggy, the mood is sad, the body is slow, and the
spirit is crushed. As discussed before, medical assessment is indicated to look for diseases and deficiencies
that can result in depression. Psychotherapy and pharmaceuticals are important tools in treatment. Movement,
nutrition, and breathwork are self-care adjunctive and
integrative therapies that can be extremely helpful.

It can also be critical to address the mind and spirit
directly in this disease. An initial look at the first Beati-
tude in Jesus' Sermon on the Mount as quoted above is
puzzling. "Blessed are the poor in spirit." "Blessed" is
translated as "happy." "Poor in spirit" means humbled,
miserable, bereft of self-confidence. How can that go
along with happy? If there is a lesson in depression, it is
that when we are at our lowest, we learn to look to a
greater power, a divine instructor, for confidence and

sustenance. Despite any or all personal achievements, the common denominator among those who have walked the path of depression is the recognition that self is not the ultimate goal.

"For theirs is the kingdom of heaven" means that when our spirit is at the lowest point, the best the Creator has to offer is ours. From a spiritual point of view, we must gain the self-esteem to accept this gift. The worthlessness and self-loathing we may feel in depression is false, and we are worthy of a spiritual gift. Self-forgiveness and recognition of self-worth are a part of the spiritual healing from depression.

Dr. Lisa Miller discusses the science of spirituality in her book *The Awakened Brain*.[1] We all have the ability to be spiritual. Spirituality can be cultivated in a faith tradition or through service, nature, or the arts. Spiritual themes within us include the ability to recognize and relate to the sacred, a higher power, and feel that we are not alone. A second theme is to share this with others.

Dr. Miller's work has also shown that while people with strong spirituality are not protected from the suffering of depression, their spiritual response and awareness is highly protective against recurrence of depression. It is as though their response to the depression is to build spiritual muscle to prepare them for suffering that may occur in the future.

Research has indicated that strong spiritual beliefs help to guard against depression and despair.[2] We can strengthen our spiritual fitness by seeking mindfulness through breathwork, prayer, and meditation. Mindfulness is a way to put things in perspective. A study of the effects of formal mindfulness meditation in depressed older adults showed significantly less depression using this strategy.[3] The formal meditation methods used in this study included Kabat-Zinn's Mindfulness Based Stress Reduction and Segal's Mindfulness Based Cognitive Therapy.[4] Other meditations may be valuable as well.

Dr. Ann Marie Chiasson's Heart Center Meditation as described in her book *Energy Healing* is a positive, affirming meditation that encourages compassion and unconditional love for self and others. This meditation helps clear the mind and focus on the heart center as the focus of healing energy for the mind and body.[5] Find a quiet and comfortable place to sit. If you want to use music, choose something calming for you. Just as the position of the hands can be helpful in prayer, the position of the hands is important in this meditation. Place your hands on the breastbone, over the heart area, with the left hand over the right hand and the thumbs touching.

There are four attributes to repeat in your mind to help focus.

- *Compassion.* Open your heart to receiving compassion.
- *Innate Harmony.* Quiet your mind and focus on being calm in the midst of chaotic things that may be happening in your life or in the world.
- *Healing Presence.* Think about your desire for healing and how you can help heal others.

- *Unconditional Love.* Receive unconditional love from God and pass this on to others who have wronged you. Forgive yourself and others.

Use this meditation—or other methods we have discussed—for five to twenty minutes at least weekly. See if the Heart Center Meditation does not affect your feelings about yourself and others.

In my own experience, I found that essential oils are beneficial in restoring my spirit. As we reviewed in Anxiety Step Four, our olfactory (smell) nerve goes directly to part of our brain that has a profound effect on our emotions. Several studies have shown some benefit from citrus essential oils such as lemon, tangerine, and bergamot, as well as essential oils from flowers such as ylang ylang, geranium, jasmine, and rose for a beneficial effect on mood.[6] Essential oils blends can be especially powerful. One blend that was particularly helpful to me contained the citrus and floral oils above. I inhaled it from my diffuser and used it (diluted) topically on a regular basis to experience a noticeable benefit.

From Phyllis

Depression is like a heavy, gray cloud, a palpable darkness, that veils the color and vibrancy of our lives. This dark cloud brings an overwhelming gloom that is real and yet often difficult to explain or to escape. I have sensed this at times, and I have watched friends and family members become despairing and depressed. *Despair* is defined as a loss of all hope. These feelings come from a variety of reasons, as Dr. Jan has already explained: physical, chemical, grief, psychological, and spiritual factors.

As a member of a faith community, I have watched other people of faith struggle not only with depression but with feelings of guilt for being depressed. They functioned under the notion that Christians were not supposed to be depressed or to have feelings of hopelessness lest they be seen as less spiritual. That way of thinking often led them into a downward spiral of depression mixed with feelings of shame and guilt.

The truth is that we all have faith. Faith is simply dependence on someone or something outside us. So, the question becomes, in what or whom will you put your faith. In other words, on whom or what are you depending? Those feelings of despair, though real, cannot be trusted. God is real. He is Truth, and He is trustworthy.

Dr. Jennifer Huang Harris says in her book *Downcast: Biblical and Medical Hope for Depression*, "Many modern Christians only depend on God to do for them what they cannot do for themselves, and as a result, God is more or less an addendum to their lives. Those who have journeyed with Him into and out of depression know they can only survive when God is present at every moment, the first and only focus of their faith."[7]

Remember Elijah, broken in spirit, prayed to die, but then he trusted God and lived. In his hopelessness, King Solomon saw life as meaningless, all vanity, without God. Even though Moses had witnessed miracle after miracle, under the weight of his responsibility he prayed,

"The load is far too heavy! If this is how you intend to treat me, just go ahead and kill me. Do me a favor and spare me this misery" (Numbers 11:14–15 NLT). Yet Moses turned to God and trusted Him. These were great men of faith who witnessed God in miraculous ways, and yet they cried out in their despair, still trusting God.

Feeling despair and trusting God are not mutually exclusive of each other. Trust that God is near even when you cannot feel Him. My friends who are deaf and use American Sign Language have a most illustrative sign for the word *trust*. It is an extension of both arms out in front of your body at heart level and grabbing hold to an imaginary rope like you're hanging on for dear life. For me that imaginary rope is the One who loves me and wants what is best for me.

I remember the morning my daughter and I sat in the waiting room while the surgeon was taking a biopsy of the tumor in my husband's kidney. I was quiet and sad. My heart was beating unusually fast, and when the doctor gave us the news we did not want to hear, I felt suddenly faint and hopeless. My tears came, and so did the question, "How are we going to do this?" My doctor friend was there with me, and she put her hands on my shoulder and gave me the best answer. She simply said, "You will do this, and you will do it one day at the time."

She was right. That is how we lived—one day at a time. I didn't have to figure it all out and fix it or fix me once and for all. I just had to get through each day.

Many days over the next few months, my foundation seemed to be shifting underneath me, and I wondered how I'd get through the day. The gray cloud of gloom was suffocating at times, and my spirit was weak, but in faith I reached out and grabbed the rope.

For some, that which is real is limited to what they see or understand or what they can prove, and everything else is imaginary. What is real to me is not limited by my inability to understand. In his attempt to describe those things which are unexplainable, psychologist and philosopher Carl Jung first used the term *synchronicity*, describing coincidental circumstances having meaning, but without a causal connection. Consider this: a man's watch stopped for no apparent reason, and he learned later that his father who lived across the country died at the exact time his watch stopped. Both circumstances were real and had significant related meaning, but how could they be explained? For those real experiences, Jung and other thinkers have seen the meaningful connection even though they were beyond explanation.[8]

Many of us have had experiences we could not explain, but often they were more meaningful than the experiences we could rationalize. For those of us in the Judeo-Christian tradition, we do not call them synchronicities because we believe they had a causal connection. They were ordained by God.

I had one of those meaningful experiences on a particular morning when I was beyond weary and discouraged. I was so weary and sad that I didn't even want to answer the phone when it rang. But when I did, it was the sweet voice of my dear friend, Jeanne, in another city. She said, "For some reason, I woke up thinking about you this morning and just decided to call you." I hadn't spoken to that friend in months, but hers was the voice of encouragement that morning as she prayed with me. Some would say that Jeanne's call was mere coincidence, but I would say that she was my rope that God provided that day.

Every day and night, I reached for the rope. Every day that rope was time alone with God, praying and reading the Scriptures. In addition, on some days, it was a conversation with a trusted friend or holding my husband's hand and remembering how God had seen us through other difficult times in our lives. Reading something encouraging or listening to a great piece of music were steady ropes. And other times, it was one of those unexplainable events, like the phone call from my friend or a perfectly timed card in my mailbox.

But the One I can always trust and hang on to is my heavenly Father, the One who provides. When I feel alone, He is always present. When my foundation shakes, He is my rock. When my spirit is weak, He is my strength. When my hope is but a whisper, He is my assurance.

Inhale

"Why am I discouraged? Why is my heart so sad? I will put my hope in God! I will praise him again—my Savior."

(Psalm 42:5 NLT)

"Spirituality is recognizing and celebrating that we are all inextricably connected to each other by a power greater than all of us, and that our connection to that power and to one another is grounded in love and compassion. Practicing spirituality brings a sense of perspective, meaning, and purpose to our lives."

(Brené Brown)

"The pupil dilates in darkness and in the end finds light, just as the soul dilates in misfortune and in the end finds God."

(Victor Hugo, *Les Miserables*)

"Thou hast made us for Thyself, and the heart of man is restless until it finds its rest in Thee."

(*Confessions of St. Augustine*)

Exhale

Pray: Dear Father, You made me to be more than flesh. You made me to be spirit too. You gave me a will, desires, and emotions. Your desire for me is that my spirit resonates with Yours. You are worthy of my trust when my foundation is shifting, and You are my rope when I cannot feel my way out of the darkness. I am grateful. Amen.

Self-Care Steps to Hope

- Practice the Heart Center Meditation this week. Notice if you have a different approach to people and problems during the day.

- As you meditate or pray, diffuse an essential oil of your choice. Notice its effects on your mood and attention.

- Look for synchronicity during the day—signs that appear to be random events but are connected by meaning. See if there is a spiritual message to you when you notice them.

- Choose one issue in your life that you will entrust to God. Talk to Him about that issue. It could be a situation, a relationship, or something your fear about the future.

Step Five

Putting Self-Care Steps to Hope into Practice

"Hope itself is like a star—not to be seen in the
sunshine of prosperity, and only to be discovered
in the night of adversity."
Charles Spurgeon

From Dr. Jan

We've reviewed breathing exercises, movement—
vigorous and moderate—foods that feed the brain to
avoid depression, and cultivating spirit as tools to
combat depression. Using mindfulness, being in the
present, in each of these will help decrease negative
thoughts and ruminations about past events and future
worries.

In Step One, we talked about practicing the Total
Breath, with Coherent Breathing, Resistance Breathing,
and Breath Moving. You can practice each of these steps
separately before doing them together. When you can
put them together, practice the Total Breath for fifteen
minutes. As you practice, simply follow your breath. As
thoughts come into your mind to distract you, just let
them go.

Find an enjoyable movement practice that you like. Vigorous exercise is great if you enjoy that and can do it. If you are already active, continue doing what you already do, and try running or cycling in a new place if you can, to see some different scenery. Try adding ten to fifteen minutes of activity to what you normally do. Remember that being outdoors and being in sunlight itself is restorative and refreshes the mind.

If vigorous activity is not enjoyable or possible for you, a brisk walk outdoors is also refreshing. If you are not active yet, check with your doctor about starting activities. Begin slowly, and build up your speed and duration. Do it regularly, and find a friend to walk with you sometimes. Companionship can cheer you up and also make it easier to walk regularly.

On the other hand, sometimes a walk by yourself can be just what you need to clear your mind. The activity and the fresh air can bring insights and solutions to problems you were worried about. You can also follow your breathing while you are moving, to work on being mindful and present. Inhale through your nose if you can, and prolong your exhale to be one beat or one step longer than your inhale. James Nestor's book *Breath* and his website (see Self-Care Resources) inform how this type of breathing can be beneficial and even improve exercise performance.[1]

In Step Three, we reviewed anti-inflammatory foods that nourish the brain and have even been shown to decrease depression. Choosing some of these may require new shopping lists and eating habits. Think about Phyllis' suggestions to try to view food as a new adventure and abundant produce as something we can be grateful for.

We covered the Heart Center Meditation in Step Four.[2] Use this meditation at least once weekly, and more often if you can. You can use the Self-Care Resources link to watch Dr. Ann Marie Chiasson's video demonstration of it. In addition to the Heart Center Meditation, once or twice weekly find a time to meditate daily, even if it is just for five minutes. Allowing a time to clear your mind of negative thoughts and worries can be helpful in getting perspective on your problems and in finding hope. If you have trouble quieting your mind, it may be helpful to listen to a guided meditation from one of the apps mentioned in the Self-Care Resources section. Meditation can be done in addition to prayer, and in fact, it may be helpful to meditate after praying, in order to receive peace and insights that you may have prayed for.

Donald Altman, a psychotherapist, developed a simple practice to help us to appreciate the present and stop the cycle of rumination, negative thoughts, and mind-wandering about our worries. The practice is called GLAD, and it involves acknowledging gratitude, learning, accomplishment, and delight in something every day.[3] The steps include:

Gratitude. What is one thing you can be grateful for today? This can include basics such as a roof over your head, food, and water. It can be personal gratitude for your work, your car, your neighborhood. You can acknowledge relationships, such as your spouse, family, and friends that enrich your life. Altman also talks about paradoxical gratitude, which is being grateful for some aspect of things you don't want in your life. For instance, if there is a job you don't like or a toxic boss, are there colleagues at work you are grateful for that you can commiserate with?

Learning. Acknowledge one thing that you learned today. It can be some fact that is interesting. It could be something you learned about yourself or another person.

Accomplishment. Identify one thing you accomplished today. It does not have to be a major accomplishment. It can be something as simple as eating healthy, getting enough sleep, completing a movement activity, making our bed.

Delight. What is one thing that you took delight in today? What is something that made you smile, something beautiful in nature that you heard or saw, a clever phrase, a thoughtful quote, a spiritual insight.

It is helpful to write these down and share your thoughts with others. This can promote your well-being and prompt others to share their GLAD moments with you.

One more thing: remember we talked about vibration and singing that stimulates the vagus nerve. In particular, low tones and words that contain an *m* and cause more vibration in the chest and body. Well, Phyllis and I thought that the song "Kumbaya" fits this bill. Don't laugh—this song has been maligned in our modern culture, with politicians ridiculing the idea of sitting around the campfire singing this song as an unrealistic, pie-in-the-sky approach to solving problems. But hear us out.

Phyllis researched the background of this song, and although the exact origins are questionable, we know that the song originated in the South as an African American spiritual. It spread to the coastal regions of Georgia and South Carolina and was sung in the Creole language by the Gullah people. Thus, we get the word *kumbaya*, meaning "Come by here." It evolved into a folk song recorded by many artists through the decades, including Pete Seeger, Joan Baez, and Peter, Paul, and Mary.

The fact is "Kumbaya" is known and sung by people around the world. Its simple and pleading melody and lyrics make it memorable. The song is a prayer reminding God that someone is crying, someone is praying, and then someone is singing. The lyrics request God's presence to come by here. The low tones and the humming consonants make for vibratory singing. I love singing and humming this myself. Try it, and just forget about the politicians.

From Phyllis

Dr. Jan has given helpful information and instruction to help ease depression, and my hope is that you will adopt some of the healthy self-care practices she recommends. I do hope one of those practices is journaling or at least writing down your thoughts from time to time.

As part of our morning quiet time together, my husband and I often read from our past journals. We read the entries aloud to each other, talk about our thoughts, and the life experiences we've had since those entries. As I read mine a while back, there was a line from a prayer that I had written that really spoke to me again: "Father, please help me to memorize the path so that I can walk it in the darkness."

That line reminded me of a scene from a novel I wrote. In this scene from *Christmas at Grey Sage*, a snowstorm strands a traveling group in the Grey Sage Inn in the Sangre de Cristo Mountains near Santa Fe. A young teacher, Emily, and Kent, a young veteran recovering from war wounds, were in the studio of that inn. Emily was drawing, and Kent was looking over her shoulder. This is an excerpt from their conversation.

"So, tell me about this children's book, or is it some secret that I'll have to wait and see?"

Emily answered, "Well, it's about a little girl named Daisy who loves flowers and playing in her garden all day long. She has conversations with the blossoms and the butterflies, and one day she asks her friend, Sunflower, what she does during the night all by herself while Daisy is asleep. Sunflower tells her that she hangs her head because the sun is gone."

Kent pulled his stool closer and looked at her drawing. "That doesn't look like a daisy or a sunflower to me."

"That's good, because it's not." She smiled pleasantly at him. "This flower is about the rest of the story."

"You're not planning to leave me in suspense, are you? Tell me the rest."

"Well, Daisy talks to her mother, Rose, and tells her she doesn't like the nighttime anymore and that she's only happy when she can see her flower friends."

"And what does Daisy's mother tell her?" Kent was almost hypnotized by the movement of Emily's pencil and watching a lily appear on the page.

"Her mother tells her to have another conversation with Sunflower about why she hangs her head. And Sunflower explains that she's been turning her face to the sun all day because that's what sunflowers do. And she's just resting and waiting for the sun to come back." She stopped and looked into Kent's eyes, which were nearer than before. "And then her mother hands her some seeds to plant right outside her bedroom window."

"Seeds, huh? This is getting suspenseful."

"Yes, seeds. And every day, Daisy waters the seeds and watches a vine grow up to her window. And she begins to see tiny white buds, but they won't open. Finally one evening, Daisy is lying in bed next to her window and looking out at the stars when she smells the sweetest fragrance."

Kent stood up. "I know. Daisy smelled cookies baking in the oven."

"Stop it, Kent. I smell the cookies too. But you're about to miss the best part."

"So, what does she smell?"

"Daisy smells a flower she's never smelled before. She jumps out of bed and goes to the window to see a large, fragrant white blossom smiling in the moonlight—her moonflower."

"A moonflower? Is there such a thing?"

"Oh yes, they're lovely, and my back garden fence is covered in them, and they only bloom at night." She showed him her drawing.

"And the moral of this story is?"

"The moral. Hmmm." She paused to think. "I'd say the moral is that nighttime comes, and we should plant seeds of hope in the daytime so that we'll have sweet-smelling blossoms in the darkness."[4]

Darkness comes, and sometimes we wait with anticipation for the light to return. So, I hope that when the light is shining in your life, you are sowing seeds of hope that you'll remember in the darkness.

Inhale

"Having hope will give you courage. You will be protected and will rest in safety."

(Job 11:18 NLT)

"Start by doing what's necessary; then do what's possible; and suddenly you are doing the impossible."

(St. Francis of Assisi)

Exhale

Pray: Dear Father of Light, when I walk in darkness, hold my hand so that I am not alone. Be my guide so that I do not lose my way on my path to wholeness, Your peace, and Your hope. Amen.

Self-Care Steps to Hope

- Practice Coherent Breathing, Resistance Breathing, and Breath Moving. Put them together for the Total Breath and practice this several times a week.
- Find movement that you like, whether it is walking, running, yoga, or something new. Make some time for movement daily.
- Check your refrigerator for anti-inflammatory, healthy foods that can lessen depression. Make a list of some things you need or want to try.
- Practice the Heart Center Meditation once or twice weekly.
- Try several essential oils and blends during your meditation or prayer time and see which work best for you.
- Use the GLAD practice to find something worthwhile in every day. Write down your responses.
- Sing "Kumbaya," and sing it with someone if possible. See if it doesn't make you smile.

Part Four

Self-Care for Grief

Step One

Take Some Deep Breaths

"Everyone can master a grief but he that has it."
William Shakespeare

From Dr. Jan

Grief. The pain and suffering we feel after a loss. While we usually think of grief after the death of a loved one, we can also grieve after the loss of a marriage or a job, after a move, or after estrangement from a friend. These kinds of losses can be one of life's greatest stressors. The often-cited Social Readjustment Rating Scale ranks the death of a spouse as the most stressful event in life. Divorce, personal injury or illness, and death of a close family member also rank highly. Notably, the death of a child was not included in this rating scale.[1]

Whatever the loss, it is important to care for yourself. Studies have shown that the bereaved are at increased risk of death and illness in the first six months to a year after the loss.[2] The bereaved are also at increased risk of cardiovascular disease, cancer, and high blood pressure.[3] This may be due to the changes in cardiovascular, hormonal, and immune systems that are likely to occur after the loss of a significant loved one.[4] The physiological changes that we discussed previously in response to stress result in increased heart rate and blood pressure, decreased sleep, and decreased immune function.[5] Especially if the grief reaction is prolonged more than six months, sleep disturbances increase risk for heart disease, stroke, and diabetes.[6] Using the strategies for sleep that we discussed in the Stress section can be helpful here. It is important to recognize these signs of stress in the grief reaction in yourself or in loved ones so that you can seek medical attention if needed and can use self-care strategies as well.

A significant potential reaction in the early days of bereavement is *broken heart syndrome* (the medical term is *stress-induced cardiomyopathy*) in which the stress response causes weakening of the heart's main pumping chamber.[7] People presenting with this problem usually have a quick recovery, but initially it can look just like a heart attack.[8]

Grief can be viewed in stages, as outlined by Dr. Elisabeth Kübler-Ross in describing the five stages experienced as a person confronts their own mortality: denial, anger, bargaining, depression, and acceptance. As Dr. Kübler-Ross herself said, "The five stages…are a part of the framework that makes up our learning to live with the one we lost. They are tools to help us frame and identify what we may be feeling. But they are not stops on some linear timeline in grief."[9]

In other words, we will experience periods of anger more than once. We will have periods of denial, bargaining, and depression more than once. We will move in and out, back and forth among these stages. What is important is that we recognize what is happening. That we recognize and face our grief where we are. Suppressing memories and thoughts of our loved ones can prolong our grief. And, at the same time, grief rumination, which is repetitive thinking about the causes and consequences of the loss, can also complicate grief. In order to recover, the griever must do the hard work of remembering and honoring the loved one they've lost, but not in a consuming way.

Ten years ago, we lost our younger son, Will, to mental illness and suicide. I have not known a grief greater than losing a child. It is indescribable, agonizing, heartbreaking. I was devastated, incapacitated, fearful. I remember the early days of mourning. What was I going to do? How could life go on without my son? It was a burden just to get out of bed in the morning, just to breathe.

One of the biggest sorrows was that I would no longer see my son on this earth. I would no longer be able to hug him. Because of my faith, I knew I would see him again in heaven. This gave me hope. And I was grateful for my faith, family, and friends. We had tremendous support from family and friends in the early days and at Will's memorial service. Our minister, Dr. Bill Nichols, led an inspiring service that was a celebration of his life; his kind, creative, and loving personality; and of the hope from our faith.

The days afterward were the hardest. As everyone else went back to their normal lives, we were left to face each day with the reality of the loss of our son. Even though our world was shattered, the world did not stop for us. How could we cope? I remember someone telling me, "Lean on God, lean on others, and just do the next thing." And that is what I did. Step by step, day by day.

While we were touched by all the kind thoughts and deeds of friends and family in the early days, I was also surprised and hurt to see that many friends and colleagues would avoid us as life returned to normal for them. I would see them duck down another hallway or cross the street in order to avoid speaking to us. Even most family members didn't want to talk about our son.

I was lucky to have some friends and family members who were willing to just let me talk and not offer platitudes about how I should be feeling. I realized, though, that most people are afraid of this kind of grief. They don't know what to say or how to act. When really, it's so simple. All they needed to say was, "I'm sorry," and all they needed to do was listen. We learned to appreciate those who were not afraid to speak our son's name and to tell us their memories of him. This was a reminder that the memory of him continued. One of our biggest fears was that he would be forgotten.

In the early days, we were not up to going to social events, and since many avoided talking to us, we learned that grief is lonely and very isolating. We so appreciated those who did reach out to us with notes and letters. I remember a letter from another mother who had lost a son, giving us some practical tips, like "Drink lots of water."

It's true that the experience of acute grief is dehydrating, due to the stress response with shallow breathing, fast heart rate, and frequent crying that occurs. I also remember the acute stabs of pain in my chest—literal heartache—when I thought about my son. It was also difficult to sleep.

Grief is exhausting.

I wish I had known then about intentional breathing. Acute grief is a state of stress, and the sympathetic nervous system is in overdrive. I would encourage those in acute grief to use the 4-7-8 Breath and Coherent Breathing to activate the parasympathetic relaxation response. It can give some relief from the acutely agitated state.

You may also want to consider a grief counselor or mental health professional early on for guidance. This can be especially helpful in dealing with guilt or regrets about your loss.

And crying in response to recognition and/or acceptance of loss can be helpful in recovery and in general is a helpful emotional release in acute grief. I think many of us have had the experience of feeling relief after a good cry. Bearing that out, research shows that most people feel better after an emotional cry.[10] The tears can actually remove some chemicals that build up in the brain during emotional stress.[11] Plus, breathing usually deepens when we cry, activating the relaxation response.

The problem may come when the crying continues even after we return to work or usual activities with others. A wave of grief may hit unexpectedly due to some trigger that we see, smell, or hear. I've realized that our culture is overly averse to tears. Crying makes others uncomfortable. I've told others that I'm not embarrassed by my tears and hope they won't be embarrassed by them either. Nevertheless, sometimes tears expressed in prolonged grief can interfere with our functioning. At this point, discuss your situation with your doctor. Neurotransmitters may be depleted, and a time of support from anti-depressants and or more intensive grief counseling may be helpful.

My parents lost their beautiful young daughter, Zee Ann, in a car accident before I was born. They had a framed needlepoint rendering of Proverbs 3:5–6 hung in their bedroom. I grew up thinking that they must have relied on those verses a lot. I never really understood their grief until I lost my son. My mother had already passed away from this earth when my son died, and, while I'm glad she was spared the grief of losing her grandson, I ached to talk to her about the grief of losing a child. I do remember something she had said about her grief, though: "You have to stop crying some time."

And, indeed you do. The grief of losing a child and of losing some other loved ones never really ends. It may help to realize that we can learn to live with it. We'll talk more about ways to remember and honor our loved ones in Step Four about Spirit.

From Phyllis

Grief. Unlike the word *happy*, which sounds light and even playful, the word *grief* itself sounds heavy and onerous. The word came into our English language around AD 1200 from the original Latin word *gravis*, meaning "weighty." Anyone who has ever grieved would agree that it is a heavy, almost unbearable emotion squeezing the life that is left. It feels like a gaping wound, oozing, leaving us to wonder if it will ever heal.

Who has lived and not experienced loss? It is indeed a part of the human experience. But so is hope. Let us look to the prophet Jeremiah, known as the weeping prophet. Jeremiah lived through some of the most tumultuous times in Hebrew history. God called him to warn His people of their coming doom. The message that Jeremiah had to deliver angered the people. Even his family turned against him. And yet, his words were true. Over a forty-year period, Jeremiah witnessed the downfall of his nation, the atrocities of brutal war, starvation, and the eventual captivity of his people by the Babylonians. He was beaten, imprisoned, turned on by his own people, and eventually taken captive himself. Jeremiah had much to grieve.

Not only did Jeremiah feel the weight of personal loss, he suffered and carried the weight of what his people were experiencing in all their loss. Jeremiah wept as he asked the questions, "Is there no balm in Gilead? Is there no physician there? Why then is there no healing for the wound of my people?" (Jeremiah 8:22 NIV). He asked the question we all ask: is there no hope from this experience?

Gilead is a real place, a region north of the Dead Sea in Israel. In Bible times, this region was noted for trees whose oils had medicinal properties. Many scholars agree that the bark was slit on a balsam tree, and the resin or oil that seeped through had healing properties. It was a valuable commodity and used for trade.

No doubt, Jeremiah knew about Gilead's balm. In this passage, the weeping prophet felt desperate for himself and for his people as they were in exile. He expressed his heartbreak and hopelessness. He asked the question, "Is there no hope? Will things ever be better? Is there nothing or no one who can help?"

Are you feeling like Jeremiah, abandoned, exiled, imprisoned by your own grief and hopelessness? Are you feeling the stress of loneliness because you have lost someone you loved deeply? Are you feeling desperate about finances? Or maybe your grief and worries are for someone else you love, not just yourself. Nonetheless, these situations leave you asking the same questions: "Is there no hope? Is there no one who will help?" Maybe like the people of Jeremiah's day, you need a balm, a spiritual balm to heal your brokenness.

I have good news. There is a balm in Gilead, and the balm has a name. His name is Jesus. He is the compassionate Great Physician and the ever-present Comforter and Healer. After years of weeping, it must have gladdened Jeremiah's heart to be able to bring good news to his people and to tell them what God had to say: "'For I know the plans I have for you,' says the LORD. 'They are plans for good and not for disaster, to give you a future and a hope'" (Jeremiah 29:11 NLT). God has the same plans for you. He is your balm of hope and your future.

Inhale

"Don't be afraid, for I am with you.

Don't be discouraged, for I am your God.
I will strengthen you and help you.

I will hold you up with my victorious right hand."
(Isaiah 41:10 NLT)

"Trust in the LORD with all your heart, and lean not on your own understanding."

(Proverbs 3:5 NIV)

"Crying is one of the highest devotional songs. One who knows crying, knows spiritual practice. If you can cry with a pure heart, nothing else compares to such a prayer. Crying includes all the principles of yoga."

(Kriplavananda)

"Weeping is perhaps the most human and universal of all relief measures."

(Dr. Karl Menninger)

Exhale

Thank you, Father, that there is healing in You. I ask for Your provisions, not those of my own. I ask for faith, not understanding. I ask for the peace, hope, and comfort of Your presence. In Jesus' name, amen.

Self-Care Steps to Gratitude

- Remember that acute grief is a state of stress. Stop and do your set of four 4-7-8 breaths several times during the day.
- Check in with a friend or family member who will just let you talk. Tell them you don't need advice, just a listening ear.
- When you are feeling overwhelmed, lean on God, others, and just do the next thing.
- Don't be ashamed of your tears. Crying is honest and can be beneficial in acute grief.
- If you find it is difficult to function when you need to get back to work or usual activities, check in with your doctor.
- Remember acute grief can be dehydrating. Drink plenty of water. (Check with your doctor to see how much is right for you.)

Step Two

Running from Rumination

"Here is one of the worst things about having
someone you love die: It happens again every
single morning."

Anna Quindlen

From Dr. Jan

One of the hardest things about the early grief was the constant thoughts of yearning for my son and the causes and consequences of his death. It was the first thing I thought about in the morning, the last thing at night, and most of the thoughts in between. Grief rumination. While this is a normal part of the grief reaction, it was so difficult to get relief from these thoughts.

What helped me was aerobic exercise. I was already a runner, and I found that taking off on a run was a way to get temporary relief from the negative thoughts. Running was something I had control over, and I could focus on the physical effort and be outdoors, both of which helped me. The physical exertion diverted my mind, and I was also distracted by the sensations of being in nature.

Swimming can also be helpful. It requires focus on physical exertion and is repetitive and rhythmic. Based on what we reviewed about the effect of physical activity relieving stress and depression, it makes sense that it could help in grief also.

For those who do not like or cannot do vigorous exercise, a brisk walk is a great moderate exercise, and it is helpful to get out in nature to feel the sunshine, see the trees, smell the breeze, and hear the birds. Just the use of all those senses is refreshing. It may also help to have a friend to walk with who can help by listening to what you are going through.

Yoga is also a good alternative and makes use of deep breathing and mindfulness. As we reviewed in the section on depression, it has even been shown to increase a neurotransmitter in the brain which is important for calming the central nervous system.

Because of the stress associated with grief, the muscles are often very tense, and it is difficult for us to relax. Progressive muscle relaxation is a way of releasing muscle tension. This activity was shown to be beneficial for relief of grief rumination in those who had recently lost their spouses, and has also been shown to be helpful for depression and anxiety.[1]

Here are the instructions for progressive muscle relaxation:

- *To begin*: lie comfortably on your back and take a few slow, deep breaths. Continue taking deep breaths throughout this activity.
- *Feet and legs*: point your toes toward your head, stretching the calf muscle, then relax. Then point your toes downward for a few seconds and relax.

Move up your legs, tightening the thigh muscles for a few seconds, then relax.

- *Hips and abdomen*: moving up your body, tighten your gluteal muscles, then relax. Contract your abdominal muscles, then relax.
- *Hands and arms*: bend your hands back at the wrist and hold for a few seconds. Relax. Make a fist with both hands and hold. Relax. Bend both arms at the elbows, tighten your biceps and hold. Relax.
- *Shoulders and neck*: Tense your shoulder muscles, bringing them up to your ears, then push your shoulders down and relax. Touch your chin to your chest for a few seconds, then relax.
- *Face*: bite and clench your teeth together and hold. Relax. Squeeze your eyes tightly shut and hold. Relax. Raise your eyebrows and hold. Relax.[2]

Take some deep breaths to finish the exercise. Do this once daily. Some find it helpful to do in the evening for relaxation.

From Phyllis

I ask again: who has not suffered the pain of loss and that deep hollow feeling that comes from being drained from sadness? What do we do to alleviate those feelings? Some of us choose to try to find some meaning or purpose in our grief and suffering. As time passes and a bit of our energy that was depleted by grief returns, we move toward helping or serving someone else who is hurting. That is often a balm for the wounds of our own grief.

Henri J. M. Nouwen, the author of *The Wounded Healer*, asked this serious question: "Who can take away suffering without entering it?"[3] As wounded healers we are to enter into others' suffering as Christ did by being available when God puts someone in our path. We are to be compassionate and to hurt when others hurt. We are to engage them in meaningful conversation that is noncondemning. We are to be tender, gentle, and patient. We are to look at their brokenness and long for their healing. In the previous chapter, I wrote about the balm of Gilead. In essence, we are to be balm-bearers.

In the midst of the pandemic of 2020, God gave Bill and me an opportunity to be balm-bearers, to engage in someone else's suffering. From our years of mission work in the Valley near McAllen, we developed a family-like relationship with a dear pastor and his family serving among the poor in the *colonias* near McAllen. Yudith, their bright adolescent daughter, became Bill's interpreter. Through the years, we watched her grow up, develop a mature faith, and get a degree in nursing. When it came time for her marriage, she wanted her father and Bill to do the ceremony.

We learned that Yudith had emergency surgery for the birth of her son, Santiago, at twenty-five weeks. When the baby was born weighing only one pound and thirteen ounces, Yudith called asking us to pray. She wept as she gave us the news, and she expressed that she had so many questions and that her faith, once strong, was now so weak.

I listened as Bill spoke to her, explaining that God had given her a compassionate, tender heart and that something would be wrong with her if she were not hurting, grieving, and asking the hard questions. And then I heard Bill say something that was deeply moving to me. "Right now, Yudith, your heart is broken. Don't equate a broken heart with a broken faith."

Don't equate a broken heart with a broken faith. Balm. Those words were balm to a broken-hearted young woman and profound for me as the eavesdropper on this conversation.

When it was apparent that the baby needed a pediatric neurosurgeon, she called again. We were able to make some connections for her, and the baby was airlifted to a large teaching hospital where he could receive the best care possible. Yudith or her husband were present with the infant all the time. His complications were many, and the care given him was excellent.

Then one evening we received the call we had dreaded. Yudith called again—this time with news that the doctors had determined there was nothing else that could be done, that only palliative care should be given. She was so weary and now faced with the decision no parent—nor anyone, for that matter—wants to make.

Yudith asked a jolting question: "Is this God's will? Are we murdering our baby if we choose to remove the life support?" We listened to her, prayed with her, and gave counsel as best we could.

Late the following day, Yudith called again. With trembling voice, she said, "I wanted you to know that our son is with our Lord." Finally, that dear girl had been able to hold her precious baby as tubes and wires were removed. She and her husband prayed over the baby and released him back to his Father. She kissed him and held him until God reached down and took him home. Yudith added, "We are at complete peace. We wondered why we had to come to this hospital if our baby was not going to make it. Now we know. It was God's gift for us to know that we did everything possible for him to be healed and live so that we would be at peace about the decision we had to make."

Such faith and such wisdom from that young woman.

If God means for us to share in the suffering, then we get to be a part of the healing too. As God's children, His servants, and His balm-bearers, most often, the balm we offer is not answers to the hard questions but the assurance of God's presence with us and the assurance of our eternities with Him. There is no better balm.

Not for a while until she has healed from her own grief, but I have a strong sense that in the years ahead as a nurse, Yudith will be a wounded healer, sharing her story to give encouragement to some other mother in the hospital where she works. Who better to identify with another woman's grief than one who has experienced it? She will tell of God's peace and His presence in the midst of a pandemic and the birth and death of her son. And no doubt, Yudith will tell them that God knows of our suffering—that He knows what it is like to watch His Son die. And she will give them the hope of eternity.

Perhaps like me in circumstances like these, you have felt inadequate as a balm-bearer. I have felt that I have little to offer anyone. And it's true. I alone have little to offer. But the One who lives in me has everything to offer; hope, comfort, peace, assurance, and eternal life.

Inhale

"The LORD is close to the brokenhearted; he rescues those whose spirits are crushed."

(Psalm 34:18 NLT)

"Grief is like the ocean; it comes on waves ebbing and flowing. Sometimes the water is calm, and sometimes it is overwhelming. All we can do is learn to swim."

(Vicki Harrison)

"Each of us has his own rhythm of suffering."

(Roland Barthes)

Exhale

Pray: Father, thank You for being near when I have needed You and for the healing You have done in my own life. Lead me to see my healed wounds as a means of helping someone else. And thank You, Jesus, for your life-giving wounds. In Your name I pray, amen.

Self-Care Steps to Gratitude

- If you find that you are having repetitive negative thoughts, try doing some physical activity. Take a brisk walk, or a run or swim if you prefer.
- Do an in-person or online yoga class and emphasize the deep breathing.
- Use the Progressive Muscle Relaxation activity to relax when you are feeling tense.

Step Three

Comfort Food

"We bereaved are not alone. We belong to the
largest company in all the world—the company of
those who have known suffering."
Helen Keller

From Dr. Jan

We were very fortunate in that many friends and family
brought or sent food to us after our son Will's death.
People wanted to do something, and this was a tangible
way to support us. It was helpful because we had family
staying with us, and we did not feel like cooking. This
was indeed a ministry to our family.

Of course, the food was comfort food. Casseroles,
fried chicken, an occasional salad, bagels, doughnuts,
cookies, cakes. We had hungry family members to feed,
and we were very grateful for all this. My husband and I
had little appetite, but we had to eat at some point, so it
was helpful that something was there. And there was
indeed some comfort in that food. Not only did it remind
us of thoughtful friends and favorite foods from traditional gatherings, but there was that instant gratification

center in the brain that recognized and welcomed the sugar and calories.

Our older son, Evan, gave a beautiful eulogy at his brother Will's memorial service. At one point, he made a side comment to Will himself: "Will, you wouldn't have liked all the attention, but you would have loved the food." Yes, he would have.

So, there was the time and place to eat and appreciate that comfort food. But, as we talked about in the section on Stress Eating, foods high in sugar and fat eventually result in the cycle of cravings that becomes unhealthy and insatiable, so we couldn't eat this way forever. After family and friends left, we returned to a healthier diet.

As with depression, grief affects people differently. Poor dietary habits are one of the negative changes in health behavior that can occur during bereavement. This may include eating more commercially prepared meals or skipping meals.[1] Some people have little appetite and lose weight. Others respond with stress eating and gain weight. Whatever the response, it's important that those grieving take care of themselves by eating healthy food. It may mean finding a meal subscription or delivery service for a while if you don't feel up to shopping or organizing the cooking. Don't be too hard on yourself as you find your way in returning to your usual routines. You have changed. This loss will affect you and how you do things. Be patient with yourself.

Remember the calming and sustaining foods we talked about in the sections on Anxiety and Depression—vegetables, fruits, nuts—especially walnuts, seafood. and lean meats. This kind of eating will lead to a calmer mind and a more durable emotional state. Grief is a physically exhausting process. Taking care of your physical body is part of your recovery. The loved one you lost would want you to take care of yourself.

From Phyllis

For me, there's something almost sacred about the dining table. I had the blessing of growing up in an era in the South where mealtime, especially the evening meal, was a ritual, and the women in my family knew their way around the kitchen. Almost at the same time every evening, my parents and my brother and I sat down to a nutritious homecooked meal and talked about the day. Mealtime wasn't something that was consciously planned, guarded, or protected. It was simply our way of doing life.

When my feet were under Mama's table, I was learning good manners and how to have conversation. I know this sounds like a scene out of a 1960s sitcom and dates me, but I long for those times again. I did not know it then, but I realize now that those mealtimes together with my family were stress relieving and life building.

Like Dr. Jan, I remember the loving gestures of friends bringing food to our family when my daddy died, and we were so appreciative of their kindness. My daddy had been in the hospital for days before his death, so we were already weary and depleted of energy. Not having to think about food preparation was truly a gift.

Somehow, as a young woman, I made it through those first few days moving through the responsibilities of funeral planning and getting Mama's house in order. It was as if I acted on autopilot, trying not to puddle in my emotions that I had safely tucked away.

I even held it together the morning after my father died. Hoping that Mama would rest a bit longer, I stayed busy in the kitchen. But Mama walked in. I could tell she had been crying, and her first words were, "Phyllis, your daddy is okay. I mean really okay." Then she explained, "Last night as I lay alone in the quiet, I could feel your daddy's breath on my neck. It was so real. His breathing was easy. It was like he was telling me he could finally breathe."

My father had died from chronic obstructive pulmonary disease (COPD), and his breathing had been labored and difficult for years. What comfort this experience had brought to her and to me.

But I remember the early evening after the funeral when the floodgates of my heart finally opened. My immediate family found ourselves together at Mama's and alone for the first time in days. I began to pull the casseroles and the salads and side dishes out of the refrigerator to serve my family our evening meal. We took our places at the table, and suddenly I saw the empty chair. The sadness washed over me like a tidal wave, and I literally got up and ran out the back door and across the driveway to Daddy's workshop. He had a swing underneath a large pear tree just outside the shop door. He would always sit in the swing, which he had made, and rest from his woodworking.

I sat there in his swing with my arms wrapped tightly around my knees and cried hard. I missed Daddy, his corny jokes, and his gentle way, and I knew sitting at that table would never be the same. There was something sacred about that table and the way we shared meals around it.

Do you just eat your food, or do you share a meal? It seems in the busy world today, more people eat on the run and out of a bag, and most often with their phones in their hands. They miss the joy and intimacy of fellowship and conversation around the table. Food is something to be shared. Think of how we observe birthdays, anniversaries, weddings, other special occasions, and yes, even funerals. Food is always involved. Food becomes a way of expressing love and compassion as we take a meal to someone who is ill or recovering or to a grieving family. Although food is a requirement to sustain our bodies, it also has a way of sustaining our souls when shared.

The Bible tells us so many stories like the story of the Shunamite woman who provided food and shelter for the prophet Elisha (see 2 Kings 4). Or Mary and Martha giving hospitality to Jesus and His disciples (see Luke 10). Or how Jesus fed the multitude with the loaves and fishes, the only miracle to be recorded in all four gospels. In each story, the Shunamite woman, Martha, and Jesus recognized the need for providing proper nourishment to the people in their company.

And then there's the story of my friend Nina. Nina was eighty-seven and living alone. She had outlived her husband and her two sons. Her grown grandchildren lived out of state. For nearly fifty years, Nina had prepared nutritious meals for her husband and family. For decades, they celebrated together around their table. But as of late, a church friend who often came by to check on her noticed Nina was growing thin.

She persuaded Nina to see a doctor. The doctor's visit revealed Nina had lost all interest in eating. Perhaps the dining table was sacred to Nina too.

There are lessons to be learned about how food provides for our needs for nourishment of our bodies and our spirits. Whether it is eating the foods that make our bodies function best, sharing a meal with a family member or friend, or providing food for someone in need, food can show we care. The way we eat shows we care for ourselves, and the way we share food shows our care for others.

Inhale

"I am the living bread that came down from heaven. Anyone who eats this bread will live forever; and this bread, which I will offer so the world may live, is my flesh."

(John 6:51 NLT)

"Food, like a loving touch or a glimpse of divine power, has that ability to comfort."

(Norman Kolpas)

Exhale

Pray: Father, thank You for Your provision of food and the way it nourishes my body and my spirit, even when I am sad and grieving. Bless the ones who grow and prepare the food I eat and the ones who express their love by the food they offer. Amen.

Self-Care Steps to Gratitude

- After family and friends have left, check your refrigerator to see what is left over and what you need to get.
- Don't feel guilty for finishing up the comfort food. Take it easy on yourself.
- Include vegetables, fruits, nuts, and lean meats on your shopping list. Ask a friend to help you if you are not up to going to the store.
- If you are not up to cooking, try a meal delivery service or get takeout from a restaurant that has some healthy food.

Step Four

They Are...Wherever We Are

"They whom we love and lose are no longer
where they were before. They are now wherever
we are."

St. John Chrysostrom

From Dr. Jan

Death feels so final. We reach for the phone to call our loved one and remember they are not there. We see the empty chair at the table. Our heart sinks at the holiday event because they are not there. We miss their jokes, their funny laugh, their warm hug. We long for one more conversation. Many times we did not get to say goodbye. The finality sinks in after we get past the initial shock of a sudden death, and also after the conclusion of a prolonged death. Many grievers say that the second year after a loss is worse than the first because the finality is realized.

My faith believes in an afterlife in which we live with our Creator who has gone to prepare a place for us (see John 14:2–3). This belief is what gives me some hope after my son died. Still, so abstract and intangible.

On the third morning after my son died, I awoke as I felt three pats on my back. I sat up with a start. I thought maybe it was my husband, but he was asleep and facing the other way. I thought maybe it was the dog's long tail, but I saw he was on the floor. I realized then it was my son, Will, telling me he was okay. This small, tactile signal that gave me such assurance, such clarity.

There were other signs in the coming days, and I welcomed them. My faith was no longer just a belief, it was a knowledge that my son was still with us. He is now wherever we are.

Writing was helpful in the early days, to express my feelings. I wrote a letter to my son. Telling him how much we loved him and missed him and that I wished I could have done more. Somehow, getting the feelings down on paper was a relief, and this expression helped ease the pain.

We established a scholarship in Will's name at the university he attended and loved. We knew he would be pleased about the idea of his memory helping someone reach their college goals. We light a candle for him at the table at special events. We remember his birthday and holidays by including food and activities that he enjoyed. He is still with us. Not in the way we would choose. But I'm grateful he is there.

Six weeks after my son died, I was diagnosed with uterine cancer. What? Where did that come from? Why now? As I absorbed this news, I found a silver lining even in this: I realized how much I did want to live. Despite the despondence after losing a son, there was reason to go on. I had people to love. I had more to do. My cancer was detected early. I underwent surgery and two years of hormonal therapy, and, despite my doctor's early concerns, I am now cancer free. Gratitude.

As I returned to work, I remembered sitting at my desk the day before my son died. I was organizing a course to improve health-care quality and patient safety. There were many obstacles. Getting the projects and participants organized and seeking support was a challenge. It seemed overwhelming and I wondered at the time if it was worth it.

Now, as I returned to those same obstacles and dilemmas, they no longer seemed overwhelming. Because it was meaningful work. I realized that it was a blessing to have work and a purpose to help others. The course was organized and continues to train health-care professionals to make health care better. And I continue to have the privilege of seeing patients and to work to make their lives better.

I experienced for myself the advice from many grief recovery books: Be of service to someone. Turn your attention and efforts outside yourself. Community participation can help to alleviate the grief of child loss and support recovery.[1] This empowers the griever and gives hope. I continue to be grateful for meaningful work.

From Phyllis

We all are walking volumes of stories, and I want to share a personal story because I believe there is much to be learned from it. In late December of 2018 after three months of chemotherapy, we were preparing ourselves for Bill's surgery on December 31. Surgery on New Year's Eve was a bit scary to me, but the doctor convinced us that we were putting his cancer in the rearview mirror and starting the New Year on the road to recovery. Looking back, he was right. But for eight days as Bill's condition remained serious, I never left the hospital. Concurrently, in the week before his surgery and the week after, we lost five longtime and dear friends. It was a very dark and sad time for us for so many reasons.

One of those friends we lost was Carol. Carol and her dear husband, Roger, had quite the love story and such a beautiful relationship. They were bright, energetic, smart, and fun people, and each of them just lit up a room without even trying.

In 2016, Carol began to have weakness in her legs and wound up at the Mayo Clinic in Rochester but returned home with an inconclusive diagnosis. By the spring of 2017, her weakness had increased, and they returned to Mayo. The doctor's diagnosis of ALS, commonly known as Lou Gehrig's Disease, catapulted them into their grief journey for the next year and a half until Carol died. ALS was not a stranger to Carol, as her father had died from the disease that robs one of all strength.

Grief doesn't just come when someone dies. Grief comes with the loss of something that you value: a job, a relationship, a dream, your health, future plans... Your normal, walking-around, everyday life. Roger and Carol suffered many losses over the next several months. Carol's weakness took her ability to walk, her independence. Her illness required outfitting her magazine-worthy home with an electric wheelchair, a hospital bed, a mechanical lift, and ramps. Her condition and Roger's commitment to help her maintain her dignity meant renovating their bathroom.

Carol was an amazing and classy lady. Every time we visited with them, she sat perched in her wheelchair with perfect makeup and coiffed hair, dressed stylishly down to matching shoes and jewelry. That was the Carol I knew. Not only was she decked out, but her house continued to be decorated with the changing seasons.

In our time together, Carol was engaging and entertaining and yet spoke honestly about her hatred of this insidious disease. She clung to the hope that the infusions her neurologist ordered would slow the progression of the disease and give her more time. It was therefore quite a gut-punch sending them to a new level of grief when the doctor told them there would be nothing to gain by more infusions. She suggested that they engage hospice.

Although Carol had hopes for the success of this treatment, her real hope came from her strong and simple faith. It took a bit of time for Roger and Carol to talk openly to each other about their feelings and their pain. Neither of them wanted to inflict the other with their deep sadness. Although Carol was confident about her complete healing in heaven, she wanted to see her grandchildren grow up, and she wanted many more years to do the things she and Roger had planned. And Roger wanted those same things and was trying to figure out how he would be able to live without Carol. And yet, in spite of his desire for her to live, his constant prayer was that God would take her before she was in pain and before she lost her dignity and that God would allow him to live just one day beyond Carol so he could attend her and care for her.

And care for her Roger did. He listened as a wise friend affirmed Roger's ability to make the necessary decisions that he would be required to make over the next months. He took that friend's advice to acquire whatever medical help was available to attend to Carol, reminding him that Carol needed him to be her loving husband and that he couldn't be both 24/7. Although Roger had help during the day, he was alone in the evenings. He wanted to be the one to give care in the middle of the night when Carol woke and was frightened or needed assistance. He wanted his hand to be the one to hold her and his voice to be the voice to console her. He was the one who loved her.

Carol, because she was Carol, made the decision to plan her funeral down to the minute details. She chose every scripture, every hymn and song, wrote her own obituary, and even chose the font and colors that would go on the printed piece to be handed to her funeral attendees. I sat with her on two occasions as she made those decisions. But Carol was not morbid about this.

Carol was accustomed to a life of serving others. At the same time she was planning her funeral, she was engaging friends and former colleagues to join her on the annual ALS walk to raise funds for research. In October, her team was the number one team in raising funds, and she had the largest team show up for the Saturday morning walk. She might have been unable to walk herself, but she motivated others to walk.

And then there was the Christmas shopping spree. In early December, hardly able to talk, Carol insisted that she needed to purchase gifts for the family and for her Bible-study group. Roger and a nurse loaded her up, even with breathing assistance equipment attached to her wheelchair, and to the shopping center they went. Carol spent half a day filling shopping carts with carefully chosen gifts for those she loved. When she got home, she called her two devoted daughters to come and help get those presents into gift bags, tagged for their recipients, and delivered to her friends. That was Carol's last external act of service. She stepped into heaven on Christmas night 2018.

Even as they dealt with such hardships, they continued to live their lives as much as possible as they always had—spending time with family and friends, serving each other and serving others.

In the weeks and months following Carol's death, we observed Roger still doing the hard work of grief. He orchestrated clearing their home of all the medical equipment and donating it to the local ALS organization so that others could use it. With the help of his daughters, he gave boxes of Carol's clothes to organizations to benefit others.

When the house was back in order, he sat down and made a list of things he wanted to do, mostly because of his desire to learn to live alone without being lonely. He visited friends who were in care facilities. He joined a ministry team for a weekend of prison ministry. He volunteered at a local nature center, guiding school groups and teaching students about birding. He stayed active in his church and joined a local GriefShare program (griefshare.org), and he set a Monday-morning meeting time with a friend who had also lost his wife.

Roger is quite the reader and historian and a lover of poetry, so he read books and decided that he didn't want to just move on as though he was leaving the past behind. He wanted to move forward because he was still alive with people to love and work to do. He became keenly aware that he would not easily graduate from one of Elizabeth Kübler-Ross's five stages of grief and move on to the next. He learned that grieving was a step or two forward and a step or two back.

When you lose someone suddenly, your grieving process is a bit different than the grief process Roger and Carol experienced over two years of living and dying with a debilitating disease. They grieved together, and then Roger was left to grieve alone.

Because I had such respect and admiration for their handling of their grief, I asked Roger this question: "What is the most important thing you have learned about the grieving process, that word of advice you would offer to someone else who is grieving?"

Without hesitation, Roger stated, "You must connect with something or someone so you know that you are not alone. For me that was my faith. I believe God's Word and that His promises are true, and then I reached out to others. If you're not a person of faith, find a person or a grief support group who will walk with you."

Roger is wise and so right. Perhaps you're dealing with a debilitating or life-threatening disease, or you're giving care to one who is. You're grieving, but do not grieve alone. Grief itself isolates and insulates. Reach out to someone so that you are not alone and that you do not feel alone. Trust in the One who loves you and wants to walk beside you. Remember, you are a walking volume of stories, and perhaps your story needs to be shared to help someone else. And when the time is right, reach out to serve, to volunteer, or to comfort someone else as you have been comforted. In serving, you have hope of healing.

Inhale

"The love within us is meant to extend outward. The closer we grow to our inner light, we feel a natural urge to share it. We all long for meaningful work, some creative endeavor that will be our ministry, by which the energies within us might flow out to help heal the world."

(Marianne Williamson)

"All praise to God, the Father of our Lord Jesus Christ. God is our merciful Father and the source of all comfort. He comforts us in all our troubles so that we can comfort others. When they are troubled, we will be able to give them the same comfort God has given us."

(2 Corinthians 1:3–4 NLT)

"A sense of meaning is the most important thing in life. That's what sustains people throughout their lives: the sense that their life has a meaning or that any particular experience has meaning."

(Viktor Frankl)

Exhale

Pray: Dear Father, the Creator of life and the Giver of life eternal, I cling to Your promises. I am grateful, even in my grief, for Your provisions. Help me trust You more and help me regain my sense of purpose. Father, I ask You to fill the cracks of what feels like my shattered life and make me whole again. Amen.

Self-Care Steps to Gratitude

- Look to your spirituality for support in your grief. Write in your journal about how your spirituality supports you in dealing with your grief.
- How have you felt your loved one's continued presence with you? Write a letter to your loved one. Tell

them what you wish you say could if they were sitting beside you.

- Think of how you can be of service to others, and make plans to do so.
- What has your grief taught you? Write it down so that you might share with someone else who is grieving.
- After you have had some time and space to reflect on your loss, review your circumstances to see if you can find a silver lining. Is there a path or opportunity that you would not have otherwise discovered? Is there a person or guide that has helped you that you would not have otherwise experienced? Is there a way you can help or serve someone that you would not have otherwise done? Write about this in your journal.

Step Five

Putting Self-Care Steps to Gratitude to Practice

"All shall be well, and all shall be well and all
manner of things shall be well."

Julian of Norwich

From Jan

I learned that the above prayer was from *Revelations of Divine Love* by Julian of Norwich in the fourteenth century—thought to be the oldest surviving book written by a woman in English.[1] It was a time of great suffering. The country was in the midst of the Black Death, the epidemic of bubonic plague that affected her region for years. She likely lost family members to the plague. Famine prevailed throughout England as the war with France continued. Julian lived in seclusion, devoting herself to prayer, and experienced a series of visions after a near brush with death. And yet, she wrote that "All shall be well." Notably, not all *was* well, but she was looking to the future and trusting in God for what *shall* be.

I survived the early days of grief with the help of my faith, family, and friends. I learned to lean on God and others and just do the next thing. I remember at times it was even hard to breathe. In Step One we reviewed making use of your intentional breathing—the 4-7-8 breath or Coherent Breathing—during these times. The simple act of taking deep, slow, regular breaths can activate your relaxation response and help calm your emotions and clear your thoughts.

And crying can help with this also. It can be a physical and emotional release to have a good cry. If you are with others, don't be embarrassed by your tears; they are part of your healing and your therapy. If you are alone, you may want to call a friend as you are able, to talk about what you are feeling, what sight, sound, or smell prompted your tears. If you are lucky, you have a couple of friends who will just listen and not offer a lot of advice about what you should be feeling or doing. If you don't have these friends (and even if you do), you may want to talk to a grief counselor, minister, rabbi, chaplain, or faith leader.

Writing is also a good way of expressing and releasing your thoughts. In Gary Roe's book *The Grief Guidebook*, he suggests a grief processing method called TWA for Talk, Write, Art.[2] First, talk with someone who will listen, or talk out loud to yourself. Sometimes, speaking words for our sorrow and our anger in a safe environment is a relief.

Next, write it out. You can write a letter to your loved one like I did. Express your sadness, sorrow, and pain in writing. Many find that writing manually with a pen on a piece of paper is most helpful, but you can also type it out on your computer if that is what you prefer. Write a poem or a story about what you are feeling. Or maybe a friend or family member has unintentionally been inconsiderate in something they have done or said. Write it out for yourself how this has affected you and see if you don't feel better. Another of Gary Roe's books, *Grieving the Write Way*, can be helpful in using writing as a strategy for relieving your grief.[3]

Finally, art it out. Create a drawing, watercolor, painting, sculpture, beaded jewelry, or craft that expresses how you feel. Focusing on creating a piece of art can help you identify your emotions more clearly, and expressing them through art can lift the spirits.

As for external supports, GriefShare has video seminars and a locator for grief support groups. And the Compassionate Friends is an international group for the support of those losing a child at any age. There are in-person support groups that can be found on their website (see Self-Care Resources). They also administrate private support groups on social media where people relate to others who have been through similar tragedies. We have listed other sources of support in Self-Care Resources.

In Step Two, we talked about movement as a productive strategy. I found this to be very useful for getting away of grief rumination. Running was helpful for me, but if you don't enjoy vigorous activity, choose walking, yoga, gardening. Sometimes pulling weeds can be therapeutic. It involves working to get at the root of something and pulling it out from where it should not be. This is hard work but can be satisfying. Find something to do outdoors, if you can, to reap the benefits of experiencing nature.

Grief is a time of great stress. As you take some time to clear your mind and meditate, do a body scan. Which parts of your body are tense, achy, uncomfortable? As you focus on how your body is reacting, you may find your muscles are very tense. The Progressive Muscle Relaxation exercise is beneficial as an overall body relaxation strategy. Too, remember that grief is exhausting, and you need to get regular sleep. You may even need to take a nap during the day. Review the sleep hygiene strategies we reviewed in Stress Step One.

Nutrition is also a part of your recovery, as we discussed in Step Three. Choose some simple yet healthy meals as you are recovering. As the food you may have received initially from friends tapers off, outline a strategy for nutritious foods. This can involve asking friends or family members to continue to help for a while, using a meal subscription service, or getting curbside delivery from a place with healthy food. And remember to hydrate. Grief is exhausting and dehydrating to the body, so you may need to drink more water than you usually do.

As discussed in Step Four, nurture your spirit. Talk or write to God about your feelings. He can take your anger, and He is with you in your sorrow. Sometimes we don't even have the words to pray, but His Spirit hears our anguish: "The Spirit helps us in our weakness. We do not know what we ought to pray for, but the Spirit himself intercedes for us through wordless groans" (Romans 8:26 NIV).

I was not able to read for a few weeks after my son's death; I just did not have the mental focus. But when I was able to read, I devoured books about grief and wanted to discover how other people handled their heartache. A book that was especially helpful to me was *Healing After Loss: Daily Meditations for Working through Grief* by Martha Whitmore Hickman.[4] I looked forward to these meditations in an accessible daily format. When my mind was jumbled and fatigued, it was a comfort to focus on these readings. I was reassured that others had experienced what I was going through, and there were positive thoughts and suggestions to relieve some of the pain.

One suggestion in particular from these readings was turning a focus to helping others. As I realized what a blessing it is to have meaningful work, the service to others became an important part of returning to function. You may find there is an aspect to your work that is a ministry to others. Serving others can take many forms, including volunteering or donating to a food bank, an animal shelter, or a refugee center in your community. If you are up to it, take soup to someone else who is grieving or who just had surgery. Helping others is empowering and can be healing.

Find ways to honor and memorialize your loved one. If they loved the outdoors, plant a tree, or donate a park bench dedicated to them. If they loved sports, find a way to contribute to their favorite team and/or fans. For lovers of the arts, contribute to a theater or a symphony. If they loved helping others, all the service contributions listed above will honor them.

You may also want to keep a few of their things in a room where you pray or meditate. Doing these things will not only honor your loved one, these items will reassure you that your loved one is remembered.

If despondence and crying become overwhelming and disabling after the time comes to return to your usual activities, check in with your doctor. Usually, they have a perspective on people who have lived through grief and know whether additional help in the form of medication or therapy is needed.

I learned to think of grief as a journey—a journey in which feelings change and I grow to adapt. This kind of grief is not something that ends. I became a different person after my son died, and I learned to adjust to being this new person. As Elisabeth Kübler-Ross and David Kessler have said, "The reality is that you will grieve forever. You will not 'get over' the loss of a loved one; you will learn to live with it. You will heal and you will rebuild yourself around the loss you have suffered. You will be whole again but you will never be the same. Nor should you be the same nor would you want to."[5]

Once I realized this, it helped me function again as a new person. I would not ever feel the grief totally lift from me; I would learn to live with it. My mother had died six months before my son. And I experienced other losses in the four years after my son died. During that time, we battled my father's dementia, followed by his death. We made decisions for my developmentally disabled and chronically ill brother, followed by his death. It was a dark time, but through each experience I learned and adapted.

I discovered that essential oils were also beneficial in managing grief. Even as I returned to work and function and began to feel better, I still had to deal with waves of grief that seemed to come out of nowhere. These were associated with a memory brought on by the season or the sight or smell of something that reminded me of my loved one. I found that an essential-oil blend of frankincense, spruce, blue tansy, camphor wood, and geranium was very helpful to me in countering these waves. One December, something triggered a Christmas memory of my son in the middle of the workday. I was on the way to make hospital rounds with a whole team of people. I pulled the oil blend out of my pocket, put a couple of drops in my palm, rubbed my palms together and then cupped my hands over my nose to inhale deeply and smell the aroma. It is amazing how this helped calm me and adjust my emotions so I could go ahead with my work. I've learned to keep this blend handy.

Finally, as you are able, share your story with others. There are other people hurting out there and they will benefit from learning how you dealt with your grief. This is actually a way to serve others. And in the telling of your story, you may find new insights into yourself as well as experience release from some of your pain.

As I learned, this type of grief is not an ending, nor does it have an endpoint. Grief is a journey, a passage, as we find the way to our new self. We will continue to have waves of grief, anger, fear on our journey. But there will also be times when we feel gratitude for the time that our loved one was with us, and when we smile to remember things that they said and did. It takes time and pain, but in grief we can find gratitude. As Rachel Naomi Remen, MD, said, "Grieving is the way that loss can heal."

From Phyllis

Grief is hard work, perhaps some of the hardest work we ever do. We are depleted of energy and desire, and we simply are not up to doing the work. But often it is work or a purpose that pulls us up and keeps us going, as Dr. Jan has illustrated so beautifully. Sometimes that work is serving others as serving gets us out of the doldrums of self.

When I was a young girl, a friend of mine was diagnosed with a rare cancer that resulted in the amputation of her leg above the knee. That experience brought many lessons for me. She was the first young person I knew with a life-threatening illness. Up until then, I considered illness and dying something old people did. And she also became the first person I knew who had lost a limb.

Probably these days, her cancer could have been treated less radically, but she went through the surgery and follow-up treatment, and then she went to rehab to learn to ambulate and to live her life differently than before. In time, she was also fitted with a prosthesis. I remember being afraid to talk to her about the whole experience, but when we did talk, I learned of her phantom pain, which is common with amputees. It is a sensation that can feel like stabbing or sometimes like needles and pins in a limb that is no longer there.

Phantom pain was once thought to be a psychological issue, but doctors now know it is a communications issue in the part of the brain and spinal cord that used to be connected to the nerves of the amputated limb. Doctors have even verified this with imaging during their patients' episodes with phantom pain. It turns out that it is very real and not so phantom or imagined at all. Some experts think that the brain and spinal cord are adjusting to the loss of communication with the missing limb. Some think it could be caused from nerve damage at the site of the surgery. Either way, this adjustment the brain is trying to make triggers the pain, letting the body know that something is not quite right.

This whole issue of amputation and phantom pain has relevance to grief. When you lose someone you love, you feel that you have lost a part of yourself—like an amputation you had not planned. You feel not phantom pain but deep emotional pain and all the questions that come when someone you love has been severed from you.

I recall a conversation with a friend of mine who had lost her husband. She was grieving hard. He had been her anchor, and now she felt afloat in a sea of despair. She was visiting in our home, and Bill and I listened to her talk about her feelings of deep sadness. Then I heard something very profound come from my husband. He said, "You've been through a most difficult few months with your husband's illness and death, and you're grieving. Consider yourself in rehab, and how long you stay there is determined by you."

Rehab is a place we go when we need help. It is designed to do what we cannot do by ourselves. Its purpose is to help people lead a healthier life. People go to rehab centers to give them tools to deal with addictions. Patients go to rehab to recover from an accident or surgery to help them regain movement, function, and strength. Cardiac patients go to rehab to learn ways to improve their cardiovascular health. There are two things that are givens with going to rehab. First, rehab is never done alone. You go there for expert help. And the other given is that rehab never changes the past. It can only change the future.

How long we stay in the rehab season of our grief is personal, but I think we can agree that we do not want to live there. Just as with an amputation, your brain needs time to adjust when you lose someone close to you. Your daily routine has possibly changed. Your conversations have changed. What used to be interaction with that person is now a longing and a memory.

If you find yourself in the rehab phase of your grief, reach out to a professional. Join a support group. Remember, you don't have to do this alone. Or as Dr. Jan did, read books that can be helpful. One book I recommend is Jan Richardson's *The Cure for Sorrow: A Book of Blessings for Times of Grief*.[6]

Like my friend who lost her leg, we must learn to live with the loss. Unfortunately, there is no prosthetic that we can acquire to replace the one we loved and lost, but we learn to adjust our lives. My friend did, and now, decades later, she is a vibrant Christian woman who has led a full and active life. She concentrated on what she had and moved forward over time.

Over the years of my life, I have experienced losses of several kinds. I have grieved in some way over each one. I have held the hands of many who suffered great loss. I have provided music at the funerals of well over two hundred people. I have witnessed grief up close and personal. I too have found that serving others has been a balm to my weary, sad soul. So often in helping others find hope and healing, we find it for ourselves.

My faith has given me strength and comfort. My faith is not about religion; it's about a relationship with the Living God who made me and who has made a way for me to live with Him forever. That brings the hope and assurance that I will once again be reunited with those who have gone home before me. I believe and trust the words of Jesus when He says, "I am the resurrection and the life. Anyone who believes in me will live, even after dying" (John 11:25 NLT). Cling to that promise.

Phantom pain is real pain. Grief is real pain. But as real as the pain is, so is the presence and the comfort of God. Lean on Him, talk to Him, and ask Him to help you accept the changes in your life. Be sure to include the Father who loves you in your rehab plan.

Inhale

"Only people who are capable of loving strongly can also suffer great sorrow, but this same necessity of loving serves to counteract their grief and heals them."

(Leo Tolstoy)

"The LORD has anointed me…to bind up the broken-hearted…to comfort all who mourn, and provide for those who grieve in Zion—to bestow on them a crown of beauty instead of ashes, the oil of joy instead of mourning, and a garment of praise instead of a spirit of despair."

(Isaiah 61:1–3 NIV)

"Whoever survives a test, whatever it may be, must tell the story. That is his duty."

(Elie Wiesel)

Exhale

Pray: Dear Father, life gets really hard sometimes, and it's not easy to breathe and move and eat and nurture my spirit. I ask for Your comfort and Your strength in me to help me move forward. I ask that you help me focus on the things for which I can be grateful, for memories, and for the hope of the future. And Father, help me to find the energy to be of help to someone else and to provide comfort to them as You have given comfort to me. Amen.

Self-Care Steps to Gratitude

- Continue your 4-7-8 breaths at least twice daily
- Choose some type of movement daily. Walking is fine. Get outdoors if possible.
- Use the Body Scan and Progressive Muscle Relaxation when you are tense.
- Make a strategy to sustain yourself with healthy food. A friend or family member could help with this. In Part Five: Self-Care Support following this chapter, we offer a few favorite recipes that are simple but comforting.
- Remember to drink water.
- Find a friend to talk with about what you are experiencing.
- Write a letter to your loved one, telling them what you would say if you could have one more conversation.
- Pour your heart out to God, or write to Him what you feel.
- Do something in memory of your loved one.
- Find a way to be of service to others.
- Use essential oils during your prayer and meditation time. Explore and find which essential oils are most comforting or supporting for you.
- Use the Heart Center Meditation at least once weekly.
- If you are experiencing waves of grief, this is okay. If these become overwhelming or do not allow you to

function, discuss with a healthcare or mental health professional.

- If you find it beneficial, you may want to carry an essential oil with you to inhale when you experience these waves.

Part Five

Self-Care Support

A Personal Plan for Self-Care

The main purpose of this book is to empower you and help you develop ways to give care to yourself when you are stressed, anxious, depressed, or grieving. These modalities of breathing, movement, nutrition, and acknowledging your spiritual nature can help ease the symptoms you are experiencing. They can also become disciplines that could improve your general well-being if practiced over time. The best news is that none of them require expensive medication, exercise equipment, or a visit with your doctor. They are all things you can do at home or even on a work break.

We have emphasized the importance of being mindful as you practice each one of these steps. Be aware of the present moment, whether you're walking outdoors or enjoying a salad. As you live in the moment and are mindful of your feelings and actions, you cannot be worrying about the past, present stressors, or concerns for the future.

We summarized all the Self-Care Steps outlined in the book in this one chapter to make it easier for you to design your own plan. Read through the detailed steps, and choose the ones that you believe would work best for you. In designing the plan, we believe that it is important to choose at least one step from each modality.

We have created a sample plan using Self-Care for Stress to help you get started. You might write your simple plan on an index card and keep it in your wallet, make notes on your phone, or use the pages at the end of this chapter. Choose whatever works best for you to remember.

SAMPLE
My Self-Care Plan for Stress

When I am stressed, I will practice these self-care steps to peace.

Breath: At least three times today, I will sit quietly and breathe deeply for two minutes. I will be aware of my breath and my slowing pulse. If I am feeling anxious, I will use the 4-7-8 breath.

Movement: I will limit my screen time for at least thirty minutes so that I can take a walk outside. As I walk I will be mindful of what I see, hear, and smell.

Nutrition: For today, I will eliminate unhealthy snacks that feed my stress and replace them with an apple, blueberries, and a few almonds. I will take the time to brew myself a cup of chamomile tea and enjoy the aroma as it steeps, and then I will sit quietly to drink it.

Spirit: I will have a meaningful conversation today with a trusted friend or family member about my stress. I will write at least three sentences about how I plan to deal with the source of my stress.

During each of these activities, I intend to be present in the moment and not be distracted by rumination of past events or worry about the future.

Now it is time to create your own plan. Choose from the following options.

Self-Care Steps from Stress to Peace

Breath

- Sit quietly with your eyes closed, following your breath for two minutes. Imagine that you are inhaling peace and exhaling your stressors.

- At least once during the day, stop what you're doing. Take your pulse and then follow your breath for two minutes, inhaling for six counts and exhaling for five counts. Then take your pulse again.

- At your next urge to pick up your phone in an idle moment, pause and take some deep breaths. Take some time to just be present in the moment and notice what you are feeling.

- Designate times to check email and social media so that you are not checking them throughout the day.

- Try deleting social media apps from your phone for a period of time.

- Try a *phast* during dinner, during a walk outside, and before bedtime.

Movement

- Do the best you can to log your screen time for just one normal day. Determine to decrease that time and increase your time outdoors.

- Take the time to take a walk in a green space and activate your senses. Be mindful of the sights, sounds, smells, and the feeling of the breeze or sunshine on your face. As you walk, give God thanks for His gifts of nature and the gift of your senses.

- Try working a vigorous exercise such as running or cycling into your schedule when you are feeling stressed.

- If more moderate exercise is for you, take a brisk walk outdoors, attempting to increase the time or distance from your normal walk.

- If you are having difficulty sleeping, review sleep hygiene strategies. Use essential oils that support sleep such as lavender, orange, or tangerine in an ultrasonic diffuser at your bedside, or make a roll-on with diluted oils to use on your pillow.

Nutrition

- Replace cookies or chips with apple slices with peanut butter, carrots or celery with hummus, berries with yogurt, or a small handful of nuts.

- Add some dark, leafy greens to one of your meals per day.

- Before you eat because you're stressed or anxious, stop. Ask yourself if you are really hungry. If it is not mealtime, try drinking water first, or take a brief walk or read something.

- Buy an assortment of herbal teas you'd like to try. Make the tea making and tea drinking an enjoyable ritual, mindful of each step. As the tea is steeping, enjoy a few moments of deep breathing as you inhale the fragrance of the tea.

Spirit

- Talk to a trusted friend about your source of stress. As you speak, listen to yourself and your friend for more insights and discernment.
- Try writing about your stress—its sources, how you respond, your ideas for dealing with the stress.
- Practice Phyllis's Scripture Scratching, copying down at least one scripture verse per day, meditating as you write.

Self-Care Steps from Anxiety to Calm

Breath

- Take five minutes at the beginning or end of your day to practice Coherent Breathing. Close your eyes, relax your hands, and breath through your nose, inhaling for a slow count of four and exhaling for a slow count of four. Be mindful of the outward, not upward, movement of your chest as you breathe, and check to see if you are breathing about five to six times a minute.
- When you feel anxious, stop, and practice the 4-7-8 breath relaxation exercise. Inhale through your nose for four counts and hold your breath for seven counts. Then exhale through your mouth with a "whoosh" for eight counts. Do a total of four of these breaths.
- As you're taking a deep, relaxing breath, close your eyes and remember that God is always near, and

recall one beautiful moment in your life. Relive that moment as you remember.

Movement

- Take a brisk walk, preferably outdoors in nature, several times this week. Be mindful of the sights, sounds, smells, and feelings you have as you walk.
- If you practice yoga, try a yoga series outdoors, weather permitting. Be always mindful of your breathing.
- If you're new to yoga, find an online video series for beginners and try it for a few days. Focus on breathing as you move and stretch.
- Try toe tapping in the morning or evening. Turn on some happy music and start with five minutes, increasing your time every few days until you're up to twenty minutes.

Nutrition

- Determine to "eat the rainbow" and see how many different fruits and vegetables you can eat in a week. Keep a food diary as you make these changes in your diet. Try to eat at least five servings of vegetables and three servings of fruits every day.
- Add a dark leafy vegetable to at least three meals in one week. Try spinach, kale, parsley, broccoli, broccoli sprouts, Swiss chard, collard greens, Romaine lettuce, or arugula.
- Concentrate on adding omega-3s to your diet by adding at least one serving of cold-water fish in one

week. Choose from wild salmon, cod, mackerel, sardines, tuna, halibut, and anchovies.

- Replace meat with other proteins like black beans, chickpeas, lentils, dairy, eggs, and quinoa for three meals in a week.

- Try new herbs and spices such as rosemary, thyme, basil, clove, cinnamon, turmeric, and ginger.

- Treat yourself to some walnuts and good dark chocolate.

- Limit yourself to one cup of coffee per day, as caffeine can increase anxiety. Replace your coffee with herbal tea.

- Make note of how this new pattern compares with your usual eating habits and how you feel eating in this new way.

Spirit

- Determine to read about the values of using essential oils, how they are made, and how they can be used. Purchase two therapeutic-grade oils for calming such as lavender, orange, tangerine, blue tansy, or clary sage.

- Diffuse an essential oil of your choice, and follow your breathing as you do. If you don't have a diffuser, just use a cotton ball with a few drops of oil.

- Find a quiet, comfortable place, and listen to a guided meditation or guided imagery, and see if this is helpful for your mindfulness.

- At least once a week, take an hour for a relaxing hot bath. Be mindful of the water and how it feels on your skin. Imagine peaceful scenes as you soak and breathe deeply giving care to yourself.

- Start your day by spending time praying and reading Scripture. Look online for Scripture reading plans.

Self-Care Steps from Depression to Hope

Breath

- In your meditation time, use Brown and Gerbarg's Total Breath, with Coherent Breathing, Resistance Breathing, and Breath Moving, for fifteen minutes. Measure your heart rate before and after. Keep a daily chart of your heart rates for a week.
- It takes breath to sing. Begin your morning in the shower by humming some low tones for the best vibration and deep breathing. Be mindful of your breath as you hum.
- Start a playlist of songs that encourage you to sing along. Choose music that will lift your spirit as you sing.

Movement

- At least once a week, make a date to take a walk with a friend—someone you enjoy and someone you trust.
- At least twice during the week, try an activity that you don't usually do. Make it an activity that involves music and increases your heart rate.
- Find a good massage therapist that uses at least moderate pressure for another way to activate your relaxation response.

- End the week with a yoga class online or in a group to stretch and relax. Focus on your intentional breathing and *ujayyi* breath during your session.

Nutrition

- Keep track of the servings of vegetables and fruit that you have daily. Aim for a least five servings of vegetables and two servings of fruit.
- If you can eat fish, include an oily fish, rich in omega-3 fatty acids in your meal twice a week.
- Replace your mid-morning cup of coffee with a cup of green tea, rich in antioxidants.
- Add berries to your diet to increase your fiber intake.
- Use nuts, including walnuts, a source of omega-3s and magnesium, as a healthy snack.
- Reduce your intake of processed foods and anything with refined sugar.
- As you prepare your food, be mindful of how the vegetables and fruit look, smell, and feel. Thank God for the variety of foods and food sources He provides.

Spirit

- Practice the Heart Center Meditation this week. Notice if you have a different approach to people and problems during the day.
- As you meditate, read Scripture or pray, diffuse an essential oil of your choice.
- Begin a journal. Record your thoughts, feelings, and things you are learning as you read Scripture,

meditate, and pray. Include your prayers in the journal.

- Look for synchronicity during the day—signs that appear to be random events but are connected by meaning. See if there is a spiritual message to you when you notice them. Record these events in your journal.

- Choose one issue in your life that you will entrust to God. Talk to Him about that issue. It could be a situation, a relationship, or something your fear about the future. Record this in your journal and refer to it often as you continue to deal with that issue.

- Start regularly doing something creative that you enjoy: drawing, painting, sewing, baking, rubber stamping, embroidery, crocheting or knitting.

Self-Care Steps from Grief to Gratitude

Breath

- Remember that acute grief is a state of stress. Stop and do your set of four 4-7-8 breaths several times during the day.

- If you find it beneficial, you may want to carry an essential oil with you to inhale when you experience the waves of grief.

Movement

- Choose some type of movement daily. Walking is fine. Get outdoors if possible. This might also improve your sleeping.

- Do an in-person or online yoga class and emphasize the deep breathing.
- Use the Progressive Muscle Relaxation activity to relax when you are feeling tense.

Nutrition

- Make a strategy to sustain yourself with healthy food and an eating schedule even when you have no appetite.
- Don't feel guilty for finishing up the comfort food. Take it easy on yourself.
- Include vegetables, fruits, nuts, and lean meats on your shopping list. Don't refrain from asking someone else to do the shopping if you're not up to doing it.
- If you are not up to cooking, try a meal delivery service or get takeout from a restaurant that has some healthy food.
- Remember to drink sufficient water. Stay hydrated.

Spirit

- Look to your spirituality for support in your grief. Pour your heart out to God, or write to Him what you feel.
- Write a letter to your loved one. Tell that person what you wish you could say if they were sitting beside you.
- Check in with a family or a friend to talk about what you're experiencing.

- Reach out to a grief support group or read one of the books we recommend.

- Find a way to be of service to others. What has your grief taught you that you might share with someone else who is grieving?

- Do something in memory of your loved one.

- Use essential oils during your prayer and meditation time.

- Use the Heart Center Meditation at least once weekly.

- When you are feeling overwhelmed, lean on God, others, and just do the next thing.

- If you find it is difficult to function when you need to get back to work or usual activities, check in with your doctor.

Summary

We hope these steps will put you on the path from stress to peace, from anxiety to calm, from depression to hope, and from grief to gratitude as you devise your personal plan. On the following pages, we have provided space for your use. However, if using a card or writing your plan in your journal or on sticky notes on your mirror works better for you, do what is best as you give care to yourself.

MY SELF-CARE PLAN FOR _____

When I am experiencing _____, I will practice
Self-Care Steps to _____.

As I take these self-care steps, I will do so with mindfulness of the moment.

BREATH: _____
_____
_____
_____

MOVEMENT: _____
_____
_____
_____

NUTRITION: _____
_____
_____
_____

SPIRIT: _____
_____
_____
_____

MY SELF-CARE PLAN FOR _____

When I am experiencing _____, I will practice Self-Care Steps to _____.

As I take these self-care steps, I will do so with mindfulness of the moment.

BREATH: _____
_____
_____
_____

MOVEMENT: _____
_____
_____
_____

NUTRITION: _____
_____
_____
_____

SPIRIT: _____
_____
_____
_____

MY SELF-CARE PLAN FOR _____

When I am experiencing _____, I will practice Self-Care Steps to _____.

As I take these self-care steps, I will do so with mindfulness of the moment.

BREATH: _____

_____

_____

_____

MOVEMENT: _____

_____

_____

_____

NUTRITION: _____

_____

_____

_____

SPIRIT: _____

_____

_____

_____

MY SELF-CARE PLAN FOR _____

When I am experiencing _____, I will practice Self-Care Steps to _____.

As I take these self-care steps, I will do so with mindfulness of the moment.

BREATH: _____
_____
_____
_____

MOVEMENT: _____
_____
_____
_____

NUTRITION: _____
_____
_____
_____

SPIRIT: _____
_____
_____
_____

Self-Care Resources

Self-Care for Stress

Step One: Breath

Weil, Andrew, MD. *Breathing: The Master Key to Self Healing.*
  Audiobook. Louisville, CO: Sounds True, 2001.

Step Two: Movement

Sleep:

  Weil, Andrew, MD, and Rubin Naiman, PhD. *Healthy Sleep: Wake
    Up Refreshed and Energized with Proven Practices for Optimum
    Sleep.* Audiobook. Louisville, CO: Sounds True, 2015.

  Sleep Foundation (website). Accessed August 19, 2022.
    https://www.sleepfoundation.org/.

  Dr. Rubin Naiman (@drnaiman). Twitter. Accessed August 19,
    2022. https://drnaiman.com.

Step Three: Nutrition

"Glycemic index." University of Sydney. Accessed August 19, 2022.
  https://glycemicindex.com.

"Mindful eating." Center for Mindful Eating. Accessed August 19,
  2022. https://www.thecenterformindfuleating.org/.

Step Four: Spirit

"Scripture Scratchings." Accessed August 19, 2022.
  www.phyllisclarknichols.com.

Nichols, Bill, and Phyllis Nichols. *Scripture Scratching Journals.*
  Dunedin, FL: GWN Publishing, 2021.

Step Five: Self-Care Steps to Peace

Nature therapy:

Association of Nature & Forest Therapy Guides and Programs. Accessed August 19, 2022. https://www.natureandforesttherapy.earth.

Meditation:

"Meditation and Mindfulness: What You Need to Know." Accessed August 19, 2022. https://www.nccih.nih.gov/health/meditation-in-depth.

Recipes:

"Recipes." drweil.com. Accessed August 19, 2022. https://www.drweil.com/diet-nutrition/recipes/.

"Tuscan Kale Salad." drweil.com. Accessed August 19, 2022. https://www.drweil.com/diet-nutrition/recipes/tuscan-kale-salad.

Self-Care for Anxiety

Step One: Breath

Anxiety:

"Anxiety at a Glance." Accessed August 19, 2022. https://www.nccih.nih.gov/health/anxiety-at-a-glance.

Breathing exercises:

Brown, Richard P., and Patricia L. Gerbarg. *The Healing Power of the Breath: Simple Techniques to Reduce Stress and Anxiety, Enhance Concentration, and Balance Your Emotions.* Boulder: CO: Shambhala, 2012. Accessed August 28, 2022. https://www.breath-body-mind.com.

Nestor, James. *Breath: The New Science of a Lost Art.* New York: Riverhead Books, 2020. Accessed August 28, 2022. https://www.mrjamesnestor.com/breath.

"Breathing Exercises: 4-7-8 Breath." drweil.com. Accessed August 19, 2022. https://www.drweil.com/videos-features/videos/breathing-exercises-4-7-8-breath/.

Matcha.com. "Dr. Weil Explains How to Do His 4-7-8 Breathing Technique." Uploaded on January 15, 2019. YouTube video. https://www.youtube.com/watch?v=p8fjYPC-k2k.

Step Two: Movement

Movement meditations:

"Yoga: What You Need to Know," National Center for Complementary and Integrative Health. Accessed August 19, 2022. https://www.nccih.nih.gov/health/yoga-what-you-need-to-know.

"Tai Chi: What You Need to Know." National Center for Complementary and Integrative Health. Accessed August 19, 2022. https://www.nccih.nih.gov/health/tai-chi-and-qi-gong-in-depth.

Yoga Is Therapy (website). Accessed August 19, 2022. https://www.yogaistherapy.com.

HealCircle. "Toe Tapping to Heal Anxiety, Pain & Inflammation with Dr. Ann Marie." Uploaded December 12, 2019. YouTube video. https://www.youtube.com/watch?v=r0aYgL_-cgw.

Physical activity guidelines:

"How Much Physical Activity Do Adults Need?" Physical Activity. Centers for Disease Control and Prevention (CDC). Accessed August 19, 2022. https://www.cdc.gov/physicalactivity/basics/adults/index.htm.

Mind and body:

> "Mind and Body Approaches for Stress and Anxiety: What the Science Says." National Center for Complementary and Integrative Health. Accessed August 19, 2022. https://www.nccih.nih.gov/health/providers/digest/mind-and-body-approaches-for-stress-science.

> Chiasson, Ann Marie, MD. *Energy Healing: The Essentials of Self-Care.* Louisville, CO: Sounds True, 2013.

Acupuncture:

> "Acupuncture: In Depth." National Center for Complementary and Integrative Health. Accessed August 19, 2022. https://www.nccih.nih.gov/health/acupuncture-in-depth.

Step Three: Nutrition

Naidoo, Uma. "Nutritional Strategies to Ease Anxiety." Harvard Health Publishing. Last modified August 18, 2019. https://www.health.harvard.edu/blog/nutritional-strategies-to-ease-anxiety-201604139441.

"Dr. Weil's Anti-Inflammatory Food Pyramid." drweil.com. Accessed August 18, 2022. https://www.drweil.com/diet-nutrition/anti-inflammatory-diet-pyramid/dr-weils-anti-inflammatory-food-pyramid/.

"Dirty Dozen." Environmental Working Group. Accessed August 18, 2022, https://www.ewg.org/foodnews/dirty-dozen.php.

Step Four: Spirit

Meditation apps (some are free, with options for purchase):

> Insight Timer. Accessed August 18, 2022. https://insighttimer.com.

> Aura. Accessed August 19, 2022. https://www.aurahealth.io/.

> Headspace. Accessed August 19, 2022. https://www.headspace.com.

Aromatherapy:

> Keville, Kathi, and Mindy Green. *Aromatherapy: A Complete Guide to the Healing Art.* Toronto: Crossing Press, 2008.

Spiritual living:

> Dr. Wayne W. Dyer (website). Accessed August 19, 2022. https://www.drwaynedyer.com.

> Kosloski, Philip. "Who were the Desert Fathers and why do they matter?" Aleteia. Last modified May 9, 2017. https://aleteia.org/2017/05/09/who-were-the-desert-fathers-and-why-do-they-matter/.

Step Five: Self-Care Steps to Calm

Lucado, Max. *Anxious for Nothing*. Nashville: Thomas Nelson. 2019.

Recipes:

> "Recipes." drweil.com. Accessed August 19, 2022. https://www.drweil.com/diet-nutrition/recipes/.

> Werner-Gray, Liana. "Recipes." The Earth Diet. Accessed August 19, 2022. https://www.theearthdiet.com/.

Essential oils supplies:

> Amazon (website). Accessed August 19, 2022. https://amazon.com.

> Abundant Health (website). Accessed August 19, 2022. https://www.abundanthealth4u.com.

> Bulk Apothecary (website). Accessed August 19, 2022. https://www.bulkapothecary.com.

Self-Care for Depression

Step One: Breath

"Depression." National Center for Complementary and Integrative Health. Accessed August 19, 2022. https://www.nccih.nih.gov/health/depression.

Qaseem, A., et al. "Nonpharmacologic Versus Pharmacologic Treatment of Adult Patients with Major Depressive Disorder: A Clinical Practice Guideline from the American College of Physicians." *Annals of Internal Medicine* 164 (2016): 350–59.

Step Two: Movement

Qaseem, A., et al. "Noninvasive Treatments for Acute, Subacute, and Chronic Low Back Pain: A Clinical Practice Guideline from the American College of Physicians." *Annals of Internal Medicine* 166 (2017):514–30.

Step Three: Nutrition

Online cooking classes:

Ramsey, Drew, MD. "Mental Fitness Kitchen." Accessed August 19, 2022. https://drewramseymd.com/mental-fitness-kitchen-register/.

B vitamins:

Lake, James, MD. "B Vitamins Play Important Roles in Mental Health Care." Last modified September 22, 2017." https://www.psychologytoday.com/us/blog/integrative-mental-health-care/201709/b-vitamins-play-important-roles-in-mental-health-care.

Step Four: Spirit

Miller, Lisa, PhD. *The Awakened Brain: The New Science of Spirituality and Our Quest for an Inspired Life.* New York: Random House, 2021. Accessed August 28, 2022. https://www.lisamillerphd.com/.

Heart Center Meditation:

Chiasson, Ann Marie, MD. *Energy Healing: The Essentials of Self-Care.* Louisville, CO: Sounds True, 2013.

Ann Marie Chiasson (website). Accessed August 19, 2022. http://www.annmariechiassonmd.com/Resources.html.

"The Heart Center Meditation with Ann Marie Chiasson." Accessed August 19, 2022. https://vimeo.com/56883155.

Step Five: Steps to Hope

Nestor, James. *Breath: The New Science of a Lost Art*. New York: Riverhead Books, 2020.
https://www.mrjamesnestor.com/breath.

Mindfulness:

Altman, Donald, MA, LPC. *The Mindfulness Toolbox*. Eau Claire, WI: PESI Publishing & Media, 2014.

Mindful Practices: Practical Tools for Daily Living (website). Accessed August 19, 2022. https://mindfulpractices.com.

Altman, Donald. "Get G.L.A.D. and Scrub Away Rumination and Anxiety." *Psychology Today*. Last modified August 28, 2019.
https://www.psychologytoday.com/us/blog/practical-mindfulness/201908/get-glad-and-scrub-away-rumination-and-anxiety.

Self-Care Steps for Grief

Step One: Breath

Kübler-Ross, Elisabeth, and David Kessler. *On Grief and Grieving*. New York: Scribner. 2014.

Step Two: Movement

Progressive muscle relaxation:

"Mind and Body Approaches for Stress and Anxiety: What the Science Says." NCCIH Clinical Digest for health professionals. National Center for Complementary and

Integrative Health. Last modified April 2020.
https://www.nccih.nih.gov/health/providers/digest/mind
-and-body-approaches-for-stress-science.

"Try Progressive Relaxation." drweil.com. Accessed August 19,
2022. https://www.drweil.com/health-wellness/body-
mind-spirit/stress-anxiety/try-progressive-relaxation/.

Step Five: Self-Care Steps to Gratitude

Grieving:

Roe, Gary. *The Grief Guidebook.* Self-pub., 2021.

Roe, Gary. *Grieving the Write Way Journal and Workbook.* Self-pub.,
2021.

Gary Roe (website). Accessed August 19, 2002.
www.garyroe.com.

Grief support sites:

Grief.com (website). Accessed August 19, 2020. www.grief.com.

Grief Share (website). Accessed August 19, 2020.
www.griefshare.org.

The Compassionate Friends: Supporting Family after a Child
Dies (website). Accessed August 19, 2002.
www.compassionatefriends.org.

Facebook groups and pages:

One Fit Widow. Facebook page.
https://www.facebook.com/OneFitWidow.

Second Firsts. Facebook page.
https://www.facebook.com/Secondfirsts.

TCF—Loss to Suicide. Facebook group.
https://www.facebook.com/groups/losstosuicide.

Healing:

Whitmore Hickman, Martha. *Healing After Loss: Daily Meditations
for Working through Grief.* New York: William Morrow
Paperbacks, 1994.

Remen, Rachel Naomi, MD. *My Grandfather's Blessings.* New
York: Riverhead Books, 2000.

Acknowledgments

Dr. Jan

I am grateful to many people for the inspiration and learning that led to this book. I thank the faculty and staff of the Andrew Weil Center for Integrative Medicine at the University of Arizona, and in particular Dr. Weil, Dr. Ann Marie Chiasson, and Dr. Victoria Maizes for their dedication and success in teaching the evidence base supporting integrative medicine. It is changing lives, and I hope it will eventually change the way we practice medicine.

I thank Dr. Rob Hromas and Mr. George Hernandez for their support of the integrative medicine programs at University of Texas Health San Antonio and at University Health. I thank Rebekah Kendrick, RN, and Casandra Chouravong, RN, Ana Vera, PhD, RN, and Charles Reed, PhD, RN, at University Health for making the implementation of our hospital-based integrative medicine program a reality.

I am grateful to Jill Sulak, LMT, who first introduced me to essential oils and helped me learn how to use them. This enriched my life and health and began my journey to integrative medicine.

I thank Thomas Patterson, MD, for all of his support and patience as I trained and implemented this new discipline in my life and practice; I am also grateful for his chef inspirations on the recipes.

I thank Frank Nichols for his artistic contributions. I am grateful to Dr. Bill Nichols for his many contributions to this project, and most of all for his encouragement and inspiration. I thank him for the oil painting lessons that helped free my mind from the pandemic and focus on writing this book. I am also grateful to Dr. Bradley Kayser and Dr. John Tierney, who helped me emerge from the pandemic and see the light of day.

I thank Leslie Peterson for her helpful editing and suggestions.

Finally, I thank Phyllis for her guidance and encouragement and for the fun we have had as fellow essential "oilers" and fans of integrative medicine modalities.

From Phyllis

I always acknowledge you, the reader. Thank you for purchasing this book and for spending your time reading it. You are on a journey toward self-care, and I hope you will invite others to come along with you.

I am grateful to Roger Boerner for allowing me to share the story of Carol's illness and his grief. Their lives and their story touched me in so many tender places.

As always, I am indebted to Leslie Peterson who provided her expert editorial skills. Not only does she know where the commas go, she was quite an encourager regarding the content and purpose of this book.

Dr. Jan Patterson, who is known as daughter, sister, wife, mother, doctor, scientist, seeker, learner, and professor, is my valued friend. She has been there to teach me about self-care. I have followed her guidance and know that it works. She has also been there when I needed her prayers. And what a gift and pleasure I've had in writing this book with her.

Without Jan and without my dear husband, Bill, I would have little to say on these subjects. Over the last ten years, I have witnessed Bill endure pain, illness, weakness, and treatment with such faith and gratitude for every caring act given to him. He has taught me much about this human journey and how to live with a healthy faith and an eternal perspective. He is a skilled listener, encourager, theologian, and source of wisdom. His love makes me a more loving person.

From Dr. Jan and Phyllis

And now to the One who made us and cares for us, we give thanks.

Recipes

Almond Toast

Ingredients

1 slice sprouted grain bread

2 tablespoons almond butter

1/2 cup fruit of choice (blueberries, raspberries, diced apples softened in microwave)

1/2 teaspoon cinnamon

Stevia to taste

Instructions

- Toast the bread and spread the almond butter on the toast. Top with fruit of choice.
- Sprinkle cinnamon and Stevia on top.
- Cut into quarters; this makes it easier to pick up and easier to eat more slowly.

Avocado Toast

Ingredients

1 slice sprouted grain bread

1/2 avocado

1 poached or soft-boiled egg, if desired

Smoked salmon slice, if desired.

1/2 tablespoon pepitas

Roasted red pepper flakes, if desired

Instructions

- Toast the bread.
- Using a fork, mash the avocado over the surface of the toasted bread.
- If desired, top with egg and/or smoked salmon slice.
- Top with pepitas and roasted red pepper flakes if desired.

Baked Breakfast Oats

A delicious and gluten-free way to use those ripe bananas

Ingredients

2 cups rolled oats

1 teaspoon baking powder

1 cup chopped walnuts (Pecans or slivered almonds may be substituted.)

1 teaspoon cinnamon

1/2 teaspoon nutmeg

1/2 teaspoon salt

1/2 cup raisins

2 ripe bananas

2 eggs

1 tablespoon vanilla

1/4 cup maple syrup (Honey may be substituted.)

1 1/2 cup almond, soy, or oat milk

Instructions

- Spray a 9 x 9-inch pan or baking dish with cooking spray.
- Preheat the oven to 375 degrees.
- In a large bowl mix the oats, baking powder, nuts, cinnamon, nutmeg, salt, and raisins.
- In another bowl mash the bananas until smooth. Then whisk in the eggs, vanilla, syrup, and milk.

- Pour the wet ingredients over the dry ingredients and stir well.
- Pour the batter into the baking pan.
- Bake for 40 to 45 minutes.
- Slice and serve. It's excellent with a compote of fresh fruit.

Note: This can be kept in the fridge for four to five days.

Spinach, Pear, and Pecan Salad

Quick, easy, healthy.

Serves 4.

Ingredients

3 tablespoons olive oil

1 1/2 tablespoons apple cider or rice vinegar

1 teaspoon dry mustard

1 teaspoon sugar

1/2 teaspoon salt

1/4 teaspoon freshly ground black pepper

1 Bartlett pear (or substitute with your favorite apple), cored and thinly sliced

1/4 cup red onion sliced in thin strips

3/4 pound fresh spinach (organic if you can find it)

1/2 cup toasted pecans (Don't skip the toasting—it adds a depth of flavor. See Note below.)

Sliced strawberries and blueberries, if desired, for sweetness and color

Instructions

- In a bowl whisk the olive oil, vinegar, mustard, sugar, salt, and pepper until thoroughly combined.
- Add pear or apple and onion.
- Place spinach on top. Toss just before serving, and sprinkle the toasted pecans on top.

Note: Toast pecan halves in a heavy skillet over medium-high heat on the stovetop for about 5 minutes until golden brown. Stir often to keep them from burning. Or you can put the pecan halves on a cookie sheet and toast in a 350-degree preheated oven. Stir after 5 minutes, and cook 3 to five more minutes. Make certain to allow the pecans to cool before chopping for the salad.

Citrusy Couscous Salad

Ingredients

1 1/2 cups vegetable stock

2 tablespoons extra virgin olive oil

1/2 cups chopped onion

2 to 3 tomatoes

2 cloves garlic

1 cup couscous

2 teaspoons salt

1 tablespoon chopped basil

2 avocados

1 cup corn kernels (canned or frozen but thawed)

2 limes, juiced

1 teaspoon sugar

Instructions

- In a saucepan, heat the stock to steaming but not boiling.
- In a separate pot heat the olive oil. Add the onion and cook 2 minutes while you cube the tomatoes.
- Add the tomatoes to the onion.
- Mince the garlic and add it.
- Add the couscous and stir 2 minutes while it toasts.
- Pour the hot stock atop the couscous. Add the salt and basil, and cover the pot to simmer on medium low heat for 8 to 10 minutes.

- While the mixture simmers, cut the avocados into cubes. Stir the corn and lime juice into the cooked couscous, along with the sugar. Add the avocado and gently mix.
- Serve immediately.

Note: This keeps in the fridge in a tightly sealed container for up to two days.

Dressing for Any Couscous Salad

Ingredients

1 teaspoon lemon zest

2 tablespoons freshly squeezed lemon juice

1 tablespoon red wine vinegar

1/4 teaspoon kosher salt

1/4 teaspoon black pepper

3 tablespoons extra virgin olive oil

Put all ingredients in a bowl and whisk. Or put it in a mason jar and shake.

Sweet Potato Hummus

Ingredients

2 16-oz cans chickpeas, drained. Reserve 1/2 cup liquid.

1/2 cooked sweet potato (or 1 small sweet potato)

1/2 cup tahini

2 tablespoons olive oil

1/2 cup fresh lemon juice

1 teaspoon kosher salt

3 garlic cloves

1 teaspoon ground cumin

Instructions

- Blend all ingredients in a food processor.
- Serve with sliced celery, cucumbers, and/or carrots, blanched or raw.

Quinoa Veggie Medley

This is a side dish you can make your own by substituting your favorite vegetables.

Ingredients

1 bunch finely chopped green onions (Or substitute 1 cup chopped onion.)

1 cup chopped celery

1 cup chopped carrots

1 cup chopped summer squash or zucchini

1 jalapeno, seeded and chopped finely (This is optional if you don't like the heat.)

2 cups low-sodium vegetable or chicken broth

1 cup tri-color quinoa

1 teaspoon salt

1 teaspoon coarsely ground pepper

Instructions

- Prepare the onions, celery, carrots, squash, and jalapeno.

- In a medium pot bring the broth to a boil and add the salt, pepper, and quinoa, stirring well. Reduce the heat to medium and cook for 10 minutes, stirring often.

- Add the vegetables and stir well. Reduce the heat to medium-low and cook for 30 minutes or until the quinoa is fluffy. Check often to see if you need to add additional broth or water. The quinoa will stick if the heat is too high or if there isn't enough liquid.

Note: if there are leftovers, the quinoa is delicious and a healthy protein added to a salad of greens, tomatoes, cucumbers, and pickled beets and tossed with your favorite vinaigrette.

Blanched Vegetables

Blanching fresh vegetables enhances their flavor and adds a little interest to a vegetable tray.

Ingredients

8 cups water

1/4 cup kosher salt

1/2 cauliflower, cut into small pieces

1/2 bunch asparagus (about 6 to 10 spears)

1 bag (about 8 ounces) sugar snap peas, stemmed

1 tablespoon olive oil

Salt and pepper to taste

1/4 cup fresh basil, julienned

(Note: other vegetables can be used, as desired)

Instructions

- In a large stockpot bring water to boil. Add the kosher salt.
- Add the vegetables one at a time, and turn the heat down to medium.
- Cook for 1 to 5 minutes
- Test one of each vegetable. When it has a slight crunch, it is done.
- Place the vegetables onto a towel to dry, patting off excess water.

- Place the vegetables on a platter and drizzle with olive oil. Sprinkle with salt and pepper and top with the basil.

Note: This can store in a tightly sealed container in the refrigerator for one week. (Keep in mind that basil does not store well in the refrigerator.) Other vegetables may be added to or substituted for the above.

Green Goddess Dipping Sauce or Salad Dressing

Ingredients

1 avocado

1 cup Greek yogurt

1 bunch fresh basil leaves

2 cloves garlic

4 green scallions, roughly chopped

Sprinkle of salt and pepper

Instructions:

- Puree all ingredients in a food processor until smooth. Taste and add more salt or pepper to taste.
- Serve in a bowl.

Note: stores in a tightly sealed container in the refrigerator for up to 3 days.

Vegetables Tossed in Olive Oil Dressing

Ingredients

4 small red potatoes, unpeeled and sliced thin

1 pound fresh asparagus, cut into 2-inch pieces (a 10-oz pkg of frozen may be substituted)

1 small sweet red pepper, cut into strips

1 zucchini, sliced

1 yellow squash, sliced

1/2 pound fresh white button mushrooms, sliced

1 7-oz jar baby corn ears (Optional, but it does add color and texture.)

Olive Oil Dressing (See recipe below.)

Instructions

- Place sliced potatoes in a steaming rack in a large Dutch oven. Add water to a depth of 1 inch. Bring to a boil. Cover and steam 5 minutes.
- Add the asparagus and red pepper. Cover and steam 5 minutes.
- Add the zucchini and mushrooms. Cover and steam 5 minutes.
- Add the corn, cover and steam 1 minute.
- Transfer the drained vegetables to a bowl and toss with Olive Oil Dressing

Olive Oil Dressing

Ingredients

1/3 cup extra virgin olive oil

3 tablespoons lemon juice

1 teaspoon lemon zest

1/3 cup sliced ripe olives (Try canned black olives or green olives stuffed with pimientos—they're both good.)

Instructions

- Stir all ingredients together and pour over the steamed vegetables just before serving.

Note: This is an excellent side dish with the Baked Parmesan Fish (recipe included).

Chicken Tinola Soup

Tinola is a traditional Filipino soup with chicken, broth, ginger, and leafy greens. Moringa contains protein, vitamins, and minerals, and has many health benefits. It can be found in some grocery stores or Asian markets. If moringa is not available, spinach can be used.

Ingredients

1 tablespoon grapeseed oil

1 medium onion, chopped

2 cloves garlic, minced

2 tablespoons fresh ginger, peeled and julienned

1 tablespoon fish sauce

3 lbs. skinless chicken legs and thighs

2 14-oz cans chicken broth

1 chayote squash, peeled and cut into 1-inch pieces
   (Zucchini can be substituted.)

Salt and pepper to taste

1 cup moringa leaves (Spinach can be substituted.)

Instructions

- In a stockpot heat the oil over medium heat. Add the onion and garlic and cook until fragrant and onions are transparent, about 2 to 4 minutes

- Add the ginger and fish sauce. Cook and stir the mixture for 1 to 2 minutes.

- Add the chicken. Stir and cook for 5 minutes.

- Add the chicken broth and cook for another 5 minutes.
- Add the squash. Simmer the mixture until the chicken is done in the center, about 5 more minutes. Poultry should be cooked to an internal temperature of 165 degrees.
- Season with salt and pepper.
- Add the moringa (or spinach) and cook until just wilted, about 1 to 2 minutes.

Spanish-Style Lentil Soup

This is a healthy and hearty soup and a complete meal
with a salad.

Ingredients

1 pound dried lentils (Flat green or brown lentils work
   well.)

1 to 2 tablespoons olive oil

1 large onion, chopped

2 carrots, scraped and sliced

4 cloves garlic, chopped

1 large potato or sweet potato, peeled and diced into 1/2-
   inch pieces

1 14.5-ounce can chicken broth

3 tablespoons red wine or balsamic vinegar

1/2 teaspoon salt

1/2 teaspoon pepper

2 teaspoons paprika

Instructions

- In a large soup pot combine the lentils with enough
  water to cover. Bring to a boil. Cover, reduce the heat,
  and simmer 30 minutes.
- In a large skillet, heat the olive oil. Add the onion and
  carrots and cook for five minutes until tender.

- Add the garlic when the onion and carrot are nearly done, being careful not to burn the garlic as it leaves an unpleasant, pungent taste.
- Stir the onion, carrots, and garlic into the lentils.
- Add the remaining ingredients.
- Cover and simmer 45 minutes, stirring occasionally.

Roasted Chicken and Vegetables

Ingredients

1 whole chicken (about 4 pounds)

Several fresh sprigs of rosemary and or sage

3 tablespoons olive oil

1 medium to large onion, peeled and quartered

2 sweet potatoes, trimmed and cut into 2-inch pieces

3 ribs of celery, sliced in 2-inch pieces

2 carrots, sliced in 2-inch pieces

Salt

Black pepper, freshly ground

Parsley, several sprigs, chopped

Note: Additional root vegetables can be added or substituted, such as parsnips, new potatoes, or fennel. Dried herbs can be used if fresh herbs are not available. Thyme can be added or substituted as a fresh or dried herb.

Instructions

- Heat the oven to 425 degrees.
- Rinse the chicken. Place sprigs of fresh herbs under the skin of the chicken. Rub olive oil over the surface of the chicken. (If you are using dried herbs, sprinkle them on at this point). Place in a Dutch oven on a roasting rack. (Use crumpled foil if you do not have a rack.)

- Add the vegetables to the Dutch oven around the chicken, and brush them with olive oil.
- Season everything with salt and pepper.
- Roast the chicken for about 70 minutes.
- Remove the lid and roast 15 to 20 additional minutes until brown and done. A thermometer placed in the thickest part of the thigh should be 165 degrees.
- Place the chicken on a platter and cover loosely with foil for a few minutes to rest before carving.
- After carving, sprinkle with parsley before serving.

Mustard Chicken with Fingerling Potatoes

A one-pan meal to be served with a salad or steamed broccoli or asparagus

Ingredients

1/4 cup Dijon mustard

1/4 cup dry white wine

2 garlic cloves

1 1/2 teaspoons fresh thyme leaves (If using dried thyme, use only 1 teaspoon.)

1 teaspoon salt

1/2 teaspoon black pepper

1 cup breadcrumbs (Japanese panko breadcrumbs work well.)

1 1/2 teaspoons grated lemon zest

1 tablespoon melted butter

2 tablespoons extra virgin olive oil, divided

1 1/2 pounds bone-in, skinless chicken thighs (4 large)

2 teaspoons salt, divided

1 teaspoon pepper, divided

1 pound fingerling potatoes, scrubbed and cut in half lengthwise

Instructions

- Preheat the oven to 375 degrees.
- In a shallow bowl whisk the mustard and wine together.

- Place the garlic, thyme, salt, and pepper in a food processor and process until the garlic is finely minced.

- Add the breadcrumbs, lemon zest, butter and 1 tablespoon olive oil. Pulse a few times to moisten the breadcrumbs. Pour the mixture into a shallow bowl or pan for dredging.

- Pat the chicken thighs dry with paper towels, and sprinkle generously with salt and pepper.

- Dip each thigh into the mustard mixture to coat the top and bottom and then into the crumb mixture, pressing gently so the crumbs will adhere. Place the chicken on one end of a sheet pan lined with parchment paper or lightly greased.

- Place the potatoes, 1 tablespoon olive oil, 1 teaspoon salt, and ½ teaspoon pepper into a bowl and toss. Spread the potatoes on the other end of the sheet pan in one layer.

- Roast the chicken and potatoes together for 45 to 50 minutes, turning the potatoes once during roasting. Cook until the chicken reaches an internal temperature of 160 degrees. The chicken and potatoes should be done at the same time.

- Serve with a tossed green salad or steamed broccoli or asparagus.

Asian Crockpot Chicken

Ingredients

2 large carrots, peeled and sliced about 1/2-inch thick

1 large red or green bell pepper, cut into 1/2-inch chunks

3 green onions, chopped, divided

2 pounds chicken breast tenderloins

2 teaspoons ground ginger

1 teaspoon salt

1/2 teaspoon ground pepper

1 16-ounce can pineapple chunks drained (Reserve the juice.)

1/3 cup light soy sauce

1/3 cup brown sugar

4 cups cooked white rice, hot

1 can drained mandarin oranges for garnish

Instructions

- Layer the carrots, pepper, and 2 green onions, then the chicken, ginger, salt, pepper, and pineapple chunks in the crockpot.
- Mix the pineapple juice, soy sauce, and brown sugar until the sugar is dissolved. Pour over the ingredients in the crockpot.
- Cover and cook on Low 4 to 5 hours.

- Serve chicken on a platter of hot cooked rice. Top with orange segments and green onions. Serve the chicken liquid in a gravy boat, if desired.

Note: This can be served over rice, brown rice, lo mein noodles, or quinoa. Pairs well with stir-fried veggies such as cabbage, broccoli, water chestnuts, onion, and bamboo shoots.

Baked Parmesan Fish

Fish and parmesan cheese? Give it a try. You'll be glad
you did.

Ingredients

1/3 cup grated Parmesan cheese (Freshly grated is best.)

2 tablespoons all-purpose flour

1/2 teaspoon paprika

1/2 teaspoon salt

1/4 teaspoon pepper

1 egg

2 tablespoons milk

4 4-ounce orange roughy filets (or tilapia)

Instructions

- Preheat oven to 350 degrees.
- In a shallow bowl combine the grated cheese, flour, paprika, salt, and pepper.
- In another bowl beat the egg and milk.
- Dip the filets into the egg mixture and then coat with the Parmesan mixture.
- Arrange in a greased 13 x 9 x 2-inch greased baking dish.
- Bake uncovered for 20 to 25 minutes or until fish flakes with a fork.

Chia Pudding

Chia seeds are an excellent plant source of omega-3s and also have fiber, iron, and calcium.

Makes 4 to 5 servings.

Ingredients

1 1/2 cups unsweetened coconut milk (or other dairy-free milk)

1/2 cup chia seeds

1 tablespoon maple syrup (or more to taste)

1 teaspoon vanilla extract

Seasonal fruit, chopped, if desired

Note: Agave syrup can be substituted for maple syrup.

Instructions

- In a mixing bowl combine the milk, chia seeds, maple syrup, and vanilla. Stir well.
- Dispense a 1/2 cup of the mixture into 8-oz glass canning jars or other containers. Cover and refrigerate overnight or at least six hours to set.
- Top with seasonal fruit such as blueberries, strawberries, or peaches.

Notes

Introduction

1. "Health Benefits of Physical Activity for Adults," Centers for Disease Control and Prevention (CDC), accessed August 24, 2022, https://www.cdc.gov/physicalactivity/basics/adults/health-benefits-of-physical-activity-for-adults.html.

2. Lisa Miller, PhD, *The Awakened Brain: The New Science of Spirituality and Our Quest for an Inspired Life* (New York: Random House, 2021).

3. Abraham Maslow, *Motivation and Personality* (New York: Harper & Row, 1970).

4. Miller, *The Awakened Brain.*

Part One: Self-Care for Stress

Step One: Let's Take a Breath

1. H. Selye, "A Syndrome Produced by Diverse Nocuous Agents," *Nature* 138 (1936): 32.

2. Cal Newport, *Digital Minimalism: Choosing a Focused Life in a Noisy World* (London: Penguin Business, 2019).

3. Catherine Price, *How to Break Up with Your Phone* (New York: Ten Speed Press, 2018).

4. Andrew Weil, MD, *Breathing: The Master Key to Self Healing*, read by the author, audiobook (Louisville, CO: Sounds True, 2001).

Step Two: Moving Away from Stress

1. "Measuring Physical Activity Intensity," Centers for Disease Control and Prevention (CDC), accessed August 18, 2022, https://www.cdc.gov/physicalactivity/basics/measuring/index.ht ml.

2. B. J. Park et al, "The Physiological Effects of Shinrin-yoku (Taking in the Forest Atmosphere or Forest Bathing): Evidence from Field Experiments in 24 Forests Across Japan," *Environmental Health and Preventative Medicine* 15, no. 1 (2010): 18–26.

3. Park et al, "Physiological Effects," 18–26.

4. C. Song, H. Ikei, and Y. Miyazaki, "Physiological Effects of Forest-Related Visual, Olfactory, and Combined Stimuli on Humans: An Additive Combined Effect," *Urban Forestry & Urban Greening* 44 (2019): 126437.

5. T. Roth, "Insomnia: Definition, Prevalence, Etiology, and Consequences," *Journal of Clinical Sleep Medicine* 3, no. 5 suppl (August 15, 2007): S7–S10.

6. Andrew Weil, MD, and Rubin Naiman, PhD, *Healthy Sleep: Wake Up Refreshed and Energized with Proven Practices for Optimum Sleep*, read by the authors, audiobook (Louisville, CO: Sounds True, 2015); Sleep Foundation, accessed August 18, 2022, https://www.sleepfoundation.org/.

7. Dr. Rubin Naiman (@drnaiman), "Heartfelt prayer is one of the most overlooked strategies for healing insomnia," Twitter, September 8, 2021, https://twitter.com/drnaiman/status/1435730283312009216.

8. X. Song et al, "Effects of Aromatherapy on Sleep Disorders," *Medicine* 100, no. 17 (April 2021): e25727; M. J. Cheong et al, "A Systematic Literature Review and Meta-Analysis of the Clinical Effects of Aroma Inhalation Therapy on Sleep Problems," *Medicine* 100, no. 9 (March 2021); e24652.

Step Three: Stress Eating

1. "Glycemic Index," University of Sydney, accessed August 18, 2022, https://glycemicindex.com.

2. "Mindful Eating," Center for Mindful Eating, accessed August 18, 2022, https://www.thecenterformindfuleating.org/; J. L. Kristeller and R. Q. Wolever, "Mindfulness-Based Eating Awareness Training for Treating Binge Eating Disorder: The Conceptual Foundation," *Eating Disorders* 19, no. 1 (January–February 2010): 49–61.

Step Four: Spirit Connections

1. Keith Chen, "The Effect of Language on Economic Behavior: Evidence from Savings Rates, Health Behaviors and Retirement Assets," *Cowles Foundation Discussions Papers* (2011): 2168.

2. Bill Nichols and Phyllis Nichols, *Scripture Scratching Journals* (Dunedin, FL: GWN Publishing, 2021).

Step Five: Putting Self-Care Steps to Peace into Practice

1. Association of Nature & Forest Therapy Guides and Programs, accessed August 18, 2022, https://www.natureandforesttherapy.earth.

2. Susan Bartlett Hackenmiller, MD, *The Outdoor Adventurer's Guide to Forest Bathing: Using Shinrin-Yoku to Hike, Bike, Paddle, and Climb Your Way to Health and Happiness*, illustrated edition (Helena, MO: Falcon Guides, 2019).

3. "Tuscan Kale Salad," drweil.com, accessed August 18, 2022, https://www.drweil.com/diet-nutrition/recipes/tuscan-kale-salad.

4. John Kabat-Zinn, *Wherever You Go, There You Are: Mindfulness Meditation in Everyday Life* (New York: Hachette Books, 2010).

5. Herbert Benson, John F. Beary, and Mark P. Carol, "The Relaxation Response," *Psychiatry* 37, no. 1 (1974): 37–46.

6. "Scripture Scratchings," phyllisclarknichols.com, accessed August 18, 2022, https://phyllisclarknichols.com/scripture-scratchings/.

Part Two: Self-Care for Anxiety

Step One: The Perfect Breath

1. N. M. Batelaan et al, "Risk of Relapse after Antidepressant Discontinuation in Anxiety Disorders, Obsessive-Compulsive Disorder, and Post-Traumatic Stress Disorder: Systematic Review and Meta-Analysis of Relapse Prevention Trials," *BMJ* 385 (2017): j3927. "Anxiety Disorders," National Alliance on Mental Illness, accessed August 18, 2022, https://www.nami.org/About-Mental-Illness/Mental-Health-Conditions/Anxiety-Disorders; "Anxiety Disorders—Facts & Statistics," Anxiety & Depression Association of American, accessed August 18, 2022, https://adaa.org/understanding-anxiety/facts-statistics.

2. "Anxiety Disorders—Facts & Statistics."

3. J. Grohol, "Top 25 Psychiatric Medication Prescriptions for 2018," Psych Central, last modified on December 15, 2019,

https://psychcentral.com/blog/top-25-psychiatric-medications-for-2018.

4. Andrew Weil, MD, "Psychiatric Medications for Adults," chap. 9 in *Mind over Meds: Know When Drugs Are Necessary, When Alternatives Are Better and When to Let Your Body Heal On Its Own* (New York: Little, Brown Spark, 2017).

5. "Anxiety at a Glance," National Center for Complementary and Integrative Health, accessed August 18, 2022, https://www.nccih.nih.gov/health/anxiety-at-a-glance.

6. Weil, *Mind over Meds*.

7. Richard P. Brown and Patricia L. Gerbarg, *The Healing Power of the Breath: Simple Techniques to Reduce Stress and Anxiety, Enhance Concentration, and Balance Your Emotions* (Boulder, CO: Shambhala, 2012).

8. James Nestor, *Breath: The New Science of a Lost Art* (New York: Riverhead Books, 2020).

9. Weil, *Breathing*.

Step Two: Physical Activity Can Decrease Anxiety

1. N. M. Batelaan et al, "Risk of Relapse after Antidepressant Discontinuation in Anxiety Disorders, Obsessive-Compulsive Disorder, and Post-Traumatic Stress Disorder: Systematic Review and Meta-Analysis of Relapse Prevention Trials," *BMJ* 358 (September 2017): j3927.

2. "Yoga: What You Need to Know," National Center for Complementary and Integrative Health, accessed August 18, 2002, https://www.nccih.nih.gov/health/yoga-what-you-need-to-know; "Tai Chi: What You Need to Know," National Center for Complementary and Integrative Health, accessed August 18, 2022, https://www.nccih.nih.gov/health/tai-chi-and-qi-gong-in-depth;

H. Cramer et al, "Yoga for Anxiety: A Systematic Review and Meta-Analysis of Randomized Controlled Trials," *Depression and Anxiety* 35 (2018): 830–43.

3. C. C. Streeter et al, "Thalamic Gamma Aminobutyric Acid Level Changes in Major Depressive Disorder After a 12-week Iyengar Yoga and Coherent Breathing Intervention," *Journal of Alternative and Complementary Medicine* 26 (2020): 190–97.

4. "Yoga: What You Need to Know"; "Tai Chi: What You Need to Know."

5. "Measuring Physical Activity Intensity."

6. C. P. Ramos-Sanchez et al, "The Anxiolytic Effects of Exercise for People with Anxiety and Related Disorders: An Update of the Available Meta-Analytic Evidence," *Psychiatry Research* 302 (August 2021): 114046.

7. "Acupuncture: In Depth," National Center for Complementary and Integrative Health, accessed August 18, 2022, https://www.nccih.nih.gov/health/acupuncture-in-depth.

8. Ann Marie Chiasson, *Energy Healing: The Essentials of Self-Care*, workbook edition (Louisville, CO: Sounds True, 2013).

9. Chiasson, *Energy Healing*.

Step Three: Foods to Decrease Anxiety

1. D. Grotto and E. Zied, "The Standard American Diet and Its Relationship to the Health Status of Americans," *Nutrition in Clinical Practice* 25, no. 6 (2010): 603–12.

2. Centers for Disease Control and Prevention (CDC), "Fruit and Vegetable Consumption Among Adults—United States, 2005," *Morbidity and Mortality Weekly Report* 56, no. 10 (March 2007): 213–17.

3. L. R. LaChance and D. Ramsey, "Antidepressant Foods: An Evidence-Based Nutrient Profiling System for Depression," *World Journal of Psychiatry* 20, no. 3 (2018): 97–104.

4. Uma Naidoo, *This Is Your Brain on Food: An Indispensable Guide to the Surprising Foods that Fight Depression, Anxiety, PTSD, OCD, ADHD, and More* (New York: Little, Brown Spark, 2020); M. Aucoin et al, "Diet and Anxiety: A Scoping Review," *Nutrients* 13 (2021): 4418.

5. Liana Werner-Gray, *Anxiety Free with Food* (Carlsbad, CA: Hay House, 2020).

6. M. C. Morris et al, "Nutrients and Bioactives in Green Leafy Vegetables and Cognitive Decline: A Prospective Study," *Neurology* 90, no. 3 (2018): e214–e222.

7. Morris et al, "Nutrients and Bioactives."

8. Naidoo, *This Is Your Brain*; Werner-Gray, *Anxiety Free with Food*.

9. Andrew Weil, MD, "Is Spirulina Safe?" drweil.com, accessed August 18, 2022, https://www.drweil.com/diet-nutrition/food-safety/is-spirulina-safe/; P. A. Cox et al, "Dietary Exposure to an Environmental Toxin Triggers Neurofibrillary Tangles and Amyloid Deposits in the Brain," Proceedings of the Royal Society B (January 20, 2016), accessed August 18, 2002, rspb.royalsocietypublishing.org/content/283/1823/20152397.

10. Werner-Gray, *Anxiety Free with Food*; P. Pribis, "Effects of Walnut Consumption on Mood in Young Adults: A Randomized Controlled Trial," *Nutrients* 8, no. 11 (2016): 668; L. Arab, R. Guo and D. Elashoff, "Lower Depression Scores Among Walnut Consumers in NHANES," *Nutrients* 11, no. 2 (2019): 275.

11. Werner-Gray, *Anxiety Free with Food*; S. K. Kulkarni and A. Dhir, "An Overview of Curcumin in Neurological Disorders," *Indian Journal of Pharmaceutical Sciences* 72, no. 2 (2010): 149–54.

12. Werner-Gray, *Anxiety Free with Food*; B. Lee and H. Lee, "Systemic Administration of Curcumin Affect Anxiety-Related Behaviors in a Rat Model of Posttraumatic Stress Disorder Via Activation of Serotonergic Systems," *Evidence-Based Complementary and Alternative Medicine* 2018 (June 2018); 9041309.

13. Werner-Gray, *Anxiety Free with Food*.

14. Werner-Gray, *Anxiety Free with Food*; "Dr. Weil's Anti-Inflammatory Food Pyramid," accessed August 18, 2022, https://www.drweil.com/diet-nutrition/anti-inflammatory-diet-pyramid/dr-weils-anti-inflammatory-food-pyramid/; A. A. Sunni and R. Latif, "Effects of Chocolate Intake on Perceived Stress: A Controlled Clinical Study," *International Journal of Health Sciences* 8, no. 4 (2014): 393–401.

15. "Dr. Weil's Anti-Inflammatory Food Pyramid"; C. Davis et al, "Definition of the Mediterranean Diet: A Literature Review," *Nutrients* 7, no. 11 (2015): 9139–53.

Step Four: Turning to Spirit

1. M. Gong et al, "Effects of Aromatherapy on Anxiety: A Meta-Analysis of Randomized Controlled Trials, *Journal of Affective Disorders* 274 (2020): 1028–40.

2. N. Zhang and L. Yao, "Anxiolytic Effect of Essential Oils and Their Constituents: A Review," *Journal of Agricultural Food Chemistry* 67 (2019): 13790–808.

3. Paul Tillich, *The Courage to Be* (New Haven: Yale University Press, 2000).

Step Five: Putting Self-Care Steps to Calm into Practice

1. "Dirty Dozen," Environmental Working Group, accessed August 18, 2022, https://www.ewg.org/foodnews/dirty-dozen.php.

2. "Recipes," drweil.com, accessed August 18, 2022, https://www.drweil.com/diet-nutrition/recipes/.

3. Liana Werner-Gray, "Recipes," The Earth Diet, accessed August 18, 2022, https://www.theearthdiet.com/.

4. Insight Timer, accessed August 18, 2022, https://insighttimer.com.

5. Larry Dossey, MD, *Healing Words: The Power of Prayer and the Practice of Medicine* (San Francisco: HarperOne, 1995).

Part Three: Self-Care for Depression

Step One: Depression

1. *Depression and Other Common Mental Disorders: Global Health Estimates* (Geneva, Switzerland: World Health Organization, 2017).

2. "Depression," National Center for Complementary and Integrative Health, accessed August 18, 2022, https://www.nccih.nih.gov/health/depression.

3. *Diagnostic and Statistical Manual of Mental Disorders*, 5th ed. (Washington, DC: American Psychiatric Association, 2013).

4. Brown and Gerbarg, *Healing Power of the Breath*.

5. Brown and Gerbarg, *Healing Power of the Breath*.

6. Brown and Gerbarg, *Healing Power of the Breath*.

Step Two: How Can I Move When I'm Depressed?

1. S. Win et al, "Depressive Symptoms, Physical Inactivity and Risk of Cardiovascular Mortality in Older Adults: The Cardiovascular Health Study," *Heart* 97 (2011): 500–05.

2. F. B. Schuch et al, "Physical Activity and Incident Depression: A Meta-Analysis of Prospective Cohort Studies," *American Journal of Psychiatry* 175, no. 7 (2018): 631–48.

3. "Measuring Physical Activity Intensity."

4. M. N. Mumba et al, "Intensity and Type of Physical Activity Predicts Depression in Older Adults," *Aging & Mental Health* 25 (2021): 663–71.

5. "Depression"; T. Kekalainen, "Effects of a 9-Month Resistance Training Intervention on Quality of Life, Sense of Coherence, and Depressive Symptoms in Older Adults," *Quality Life Research* 27 (2018): 455–65.

6. "Low-Back Pain and Complementary Health Approaches: What You Need to Know," National Center for Complementary and Integrative Health, accessed August 18, 2022, https://www.nccih.nih.gov/health/low-back-pain-and-complementary-health-approaches-what-you-need-to-know; Z. Huan et al, "Systematic Review and Meta-Analysis: Tai Chi for Preventing Falls in Older Adults," *BMJ Open* 7, no. 2 (February 6, 2017): e013661.

7. C. C. Streeter et al, "Treatment of Major Depressive Disorder with Iyengar Yoga and Coherent Breathing: A Randomized Controlled Dosing Study," *Journal of Alternative and Complementary Medicine* 23, no. 3 (2017): 201–07.

8. Streeter et al, "Thalamic Gamma Aminobutyric Acid Level."

9. T. Field, "Massage Therapy Research Review," *Complementary Therapies in Clinical Practice*. 20, no. 4 (2014): 224–29.

Step Three: Are You What You Eat?

1. Jean Anthelme Brillat-Savarin, *The Physiology of Taste: Or Meditations on Transcendental Gastronomy*, trans. M. F. K. Fisher (New York: Vintage, 2011).

2. I. Lazarevich et al, "Depression and Food Consumption in Mexican College Students," *Nutricion Hospitalaria* 35, no. 3 (2018): 620–26; H. M. Francis et al, "A Brief Diet Intervention Can Reduce Symptoms of Depression in Young Adults: A Randomized Controlled Trial," *PLoS ONE* 14, no. 10 (2019): e0222768.

3. P. N. Arfirsta Dharmayani et al, "Association Between Fruit and Vegetable Consumption and Depression Symptoms in Young People and Adults Aged 15–45: A Systematic Review of Cohort Studies," *International Journal of Environmental Research and Public Health* 18 (2021): 780; Y. Yang, Y. Kim and Y. Je. "Fish Consumption and Risk of Depression: Epidemiological Evidence from Prospective Studies," *Asia-Pacific Psychiatry* 10, no. 4 (2018): e12335.

4. O. I. Okereke et al, "Effect of Long-Term Supplementation with Marine Omega-3 Fatty Acids vs Placebo on Risk of Depression or Clinically Relevant Depressive Symptoms and on Change in Mood Scores: A Randomized Clinical Trial," *Journal of the American Medical Association* 326, no. 23 (December 21, 2021): 2385–94.

5. C. Davis et al, "Definition of the Mediterranean Diet."

6. N. Parletta et al, "A Mediterranean-Style Dietary Intervention Supplemented with Fish Oil Improves Diet Quality and Mental Health in People with Depression: A Randomized Controlled Trial," *Nutritional Neuroscience* 22, no. 7 (2019): 474–87; A. Sanchez Villegas et al, "Association of the Mediterranean Dietary Pattern with the Incidence of Depression: The Seguimiento Universidad de Navarra/University of Navarra Follow-Up (SUN) Cohort," *Archives of General Psychiatry* 66 (2009): 1090–98.

7. T. Psaltopoulou et al, "Mediterranean Diet, Stroke, Cognitive Impairment, and Depression: A Meta-Analysis," *Annals of Neurology*

74 (2013): 580–91; A. Ventriglio et al, "Mediterranean Diet and Its Benefits on Health and Mental Health: A Literature Review," *Clinical Practice & Epidemiology in Mental Health* 16, suppl-1, M11 (2020): 156–64.

8. "Dr. Weil's Anti-Inflammatory Food Pyramid."

9. S. E. Jackson et al, "Is There a Relationship Between Chocolate Consumption and Symptoms of Depression? A Cross-Sectional Survey of 13,626 US Adults," *Depression and Anxiety* 36, no. 10 (2019): 987–95.

10. "The American Heart Association Diet and Lifestyle Recommendations," American Heart Association, accessed August 18, 2022, https://www.heart.org/en/healthy-living/healthy-eating/eat-smart/nutrition-basics/aha-diet-and-lifestyle-recommendations.

11. K. Mikkelsen, L. Stojanovska and V. Apostolopoulos, "The Effects of Vitamin B in Depression," *Current Medicinal Chemistry* 23, no. 38 (2016): 4317–37.

12. A. Bender, K. E. Hagan and N. Kingston, "The Association of Folate and Depression: A Meta-Analysis," *Journal of Psychiatric Research* 95 (2017): 9–18.

13. A. M. Hvas et al, "Vitamin B6 Level Is Associated with Symptoms of Depression," *Psychotherapy and Psychosomatics* 73, no. 6 (2004): 340–43; E. U. Syed, M. Wasay and S. Awan, "Vitamin B12 Supplementation in Treating Major Depressive Disorder: A Randomized Controlled Trial," *Open Neurology Journal* 7 (2013): 44–48; J. G. Walker et al, "Oral Folic Acid and Vitamin B-12 Supplementation to Prevent Cognitive Decline in Community-Dwelling Older Adults with Depressive Symptoms—the Beyond Ageing Project: A Randomized Controlled Trial," *American Journal of Clinical Nutrition* 95, no. 1 (2012): 194–203.

14. M. Kaviani et al, "Effects of Vitamin D Supplementation on Depression and Some Involved Neurotransmitters," *Journal of Affective Disorders* 269 (2020): 28–35.

15. A. Fonte and B. Coutinho, "Seasonal Sensitivity and Psychiatric Morbidity: Study about Seasonal Affective Disorder," *BMC Psychiatry* 21 (2021): 317; A. E. Stewart et al, "Possible Contributions of Skin Pigmentation and Vitamin D in a Polyfactorial Model of Seasonal Effective Disorder," *Medical Hypotheses* 83 (2014): 517–25.

16. J. A. Pasco et al, "Dietary Selenium and Major Depression: A Nested Case-Control Study," *Complementary Therapies in Medicine* 20 (2012): 119–23.

17. A. Khodavirdipour, F. Haddadi and S. Keshavarzi, "Chromium Supplementation; Negotiation with Diabetes Mellitus, Hyperlipidemia, and Depression," *Journal of Diabetes & Metabolic Disorders* 19 (2020): 585–95.

18. Francis et al, "A Brief Diet Intervention."

19. A. Shamsi-Goushki et al, "Effects of High White and Brown Sugar Consumption on Serum Level of Brain-Derived Neurotrophic Factor, Insulin Resistance, and Body Weight in Albino Rats," *Journal of Obesity & Metabolic Syndrome* 29 (2020): 320–24.

20. J. Gilbert et al, "Current Understanding of the Human Microbiome," *Nature Medicine* 24, no. 4 (2018): 392–400; J. A. Foster and K. M. Neufeld, "Gut-Brain Axis: How the Microbiome Influences Anxiety and Depression," *Trends in Neurosciences* 36, no. 5 (2013): 305.

21. Foster and Neufeld, "Gut-brain axis"; Y. Kim and C. Shin, "The Microbiota-Gut-Brain Axis in Neuropsychiatric Disorders: Pathophysiological Mechanisms and Novel Treatments," *Current Neuropharmacology* 16 (2018): 559–73.

22. H. Jiang et al, "Altered Fecal Microbiota Composition in Patients with Major Depressive Disorder," *Brain, Behavior, and Immunity* 48 (2015): 186–94; P. Zheng et al, "Gut Microbiome Remodeling Induces

Depressive-Like Behaviors Through a Pathway Mediated by the Host's Metabolism," *Molecular Psychiatry* 21 (2016): 786–96.

23. D. McDonald et al, "American Gut: An Open Platform for Citizen Science Microbiome Research," *mSystems* 3, no. 3 (2018): e00031–18.

24. S. J. Yong et al, "Antidepressive Mechanisms of Probiotics and Their Therapeutic Potential," *Frontiers Neuroscience* 13 (2020): 1362; C. J. K. Wallace and R. Milev, "The Effects of Probiotics on Depressive Symptoms in Humans: A Systematic Review," *Annals of General Psychiatry* 16 (2017): 14.

25. Yong et al, "Antidepressive mechanisms."

26. Yong et al, "Antidepressive mechanisms"; Wallace and Milev, "The Effects of probiotics."

27. Yong et al, "Antidepressive mechanisms."

Step Four: The Poor in Spirit

1. Miller, *The Awakened Brain.*

2. Miller, *The Awakened Brain.*

3. J. Kabat-Zinn, "An Outpatient Program in Behavioral Medicine for Chronic Pain Patients Based on the Practice of Mindfulness Meditation: Theoretical Considerations and Preliminary Results," *General Hospital Psychiatry* 4, no. 1 (April 1982): 33–47.

4. Z. V. Segal, J. M. G. Williams and J. D. Teasdale, *Mindfulness-Based Cognitive Therapy for Depression* (New York: Guilford Press, 2012).

5. Chiasson, *Energy Healing.*

6. D. P. DeSousa et al, "Essential Oils and Their Constituents: An Alternative Source for Novel Antidepressants," *Molecules* 22 (2017):

1290; X. Han et al, "Bergamot (*Citrus bergamia*) Essential Oil Inhalation Improves Positive Feelings in the Waiting Room of a Mental Health Treatment Center: A Pilot Study, *Phytotherapy Research* 31 (2017): 812–16.

7. Jennifer Huang Harris, MD, Harold Koenig, MD, and John Peteet, MD, *Downcast: Biblical and Medical Hope for Depression* (Bristol, TN: Christian Medical and Dental Association, 2021).

8. C. J. Yung, *Synchronicity: An Acausal Connecting Principle*, trans. R. F. C. Hull, from vol. 8 of the *Collected Works of C. J. Jung* (Princeton: Princeton University Press, 2010).

Step Five: Putting Self-Care Steps to Hope into Practice

1. Nestor, *Breath*.

2. Chiasson, *Energy Healing*.

3. Donald Altman, MA, LPC, *The Mindfulness Toolbox* (Eau Claire, WI: PESI Publishing & Media, 2014).

4. Phyllis Clark Nichols, *Christmas at Grey Sage* (Grand Rapids: Gilead Publishing, 2017).

Part Four: Self-Care for Grief

Step One: Taking Some Deep Breaths

1. T. H. Holmes and R. H. Rahe, "The Social Readjustment Rating Scale," *Journal of Psychosomatic Research* 11 (1967): 213–18.

2. T. Buckley et al, "Physiological Correlates of Bereavement and the Impact of Bereavement Interventions," *Dialogues in Clinical Neuroscience* 14 (2012): 129–39; E. Mostofsky et al, "Risk of Acute Myocardial Infarction after the Death of a Significant Person in One's

Life," *Circulation* 125 (2012): 491–96; M. Stoebe, H. Schut and W. Stroebe, "Health Outcomes of Bereavement," *Lancet* 370 (2007): 1960–73.

3. M. O'Connor, "Grief: A Brief History of Research on How Body, Mind, and Brain Adapt," *Psychosomatic Medicine* 81 (2019): 731–38.

4. E. Mostofsky et al, "Risk of Acute Myocardial Infarction"; C. P. Fagundes and E. L. Wu, "Matters of the Heart: Grief, Morbidity, and Mortality," *Current Directions in Psychological Science* 29 (2020): 235–41; T. M. Mason and A. R. Duffy, "Complicated Grief and Cortisol Response: An Integrative Review of the Literature," *Journal of the American Psychiatric Nurses Association* 25 (2019): 181–88.

5. E. Mostofsky et al, "Risk of Acute Myocardial Infarction"; M. Stoebe, H. Schut and W. Stroebe, "Health Outcomes of Bereavement."

6. K. L. Szuhany et al, "Impact of Sleep on Complicated Grief Severity and Outcomes," *Depression and Anxiety* 37 (2020): 73–80.

7. L. Zhang and I. Pina, "Stress-Induced Cardiomyopathy," *Heart Failure Clinics* 15 (2019): 41–53.

8. M. Stoebe, H. Schut and W. Stroebe, "Health outcomes of bereavement"; A. Prasad, A. Lerman and C. S. Rihal, "Apical Ballooning Syndrome (Tako-Tsubo or Stress Cardiomyopathy): A Mimic of Acute Myocardial Infarction," *American Heart Journal* 155 (2008): 408–17; L. Zhang and I. Pina, "Stress-Induced Cardiomyopathy."

9. Elisabeth Kübler-Ross, *On Death and Dying* (New York: Macmillan, 1973); Elisabeth Kübler-Ross and David Kessler, *On Grief and Grieving* (New York: Scribner, 2014).

10. A. Gracanin, L. M. Bylsma and A. J. J. M. Vinghoets, "Is Crying a Self-Soothing Behavior?" *Frontiers in Psychology* 18, no. 5 (2014): 502.

11. W. H. Frey et al, "Effect of Stimulus on the Chemical Composition of Human Tears," *American Journal of Ophthalmology* 92

(1981): 559–67; William H. Frey with Muriel Langseth, *Crying: The Mystery of Tears* (Minneapolis: Winston Press and Harper & Row, 1985).

Step Two: Running from Rumination

1. L. M. Knowles et al, "A Controlled Trial of Two Mind-Body Interventions for Grief in Widows and Widowers," *Journal of Consulting and Clinical Psychology* 89 (2021): 640–47; M. P. Twohig et al, "A Randomized Clinical Trial of Acceptance and Commitment Therapy Versus Progressive Relaxation Training for Obsessive-Compulsive Disorder," *Journal of Consulting and Clinical Psychology* 78, no. 5 (2010): 705–16; P. Klainin-Yobas et al, "Effects of Relaxation Interventions on Depression and Anxiety Among Older Adults: A Systemic Review," *Aging & Mental Health* 19 (2015): 1043–55.

2. "Mind and Body Approaches for Stress and Anxiety: What the Science Says," National Center for Complementary and Integrative Health, last modified April 2020, https://www.nccih.nih.gov/health/providers/digest/mind-and-body-approaches-for-stress-science; "Try Progressive Relaxation," drweil.com, accessed August 18, 2022, https://www.drweil.com/health-wellness/body-mind-spirit/stress-anxiety/try-progressive-relaxation/.

3. Henri J. M. Nouwen, *The Wounded Healer: Ministry in Contemporary Society* (New York: Doubleday, 1972).

Step Three: Comfort Food

1. C. P. Fagundes, "Matters of the Heart."

Step Four: They Are...Wherever We Are

1. X. Zhao et al. "What Are the Long-Term Effects of Child Loss on Parental Health? Social Integration as Mediator," *Comprehensive Psychiatry* 100 (2020): 15282.

Step Five: Putting Self–Care Steps to Gratitude into Practice

1. Julian of Norwich, *Revelations of Divine Love* (independently published, 2021).

2. Gary Roe, *The Grief Guidebook* (self-pub., 2021).

3. Gary Roe, *Grieving the Write Way Journal and Workbook* (self-pub., 2021).

4. Martha Whitmore Hickman, *Healing After Loss: Daily Meditations for Working Through Grief* (New York: William Morrow Paperbacks, 1994).

5. Kübler-Ross and Kessler, *On Grief and Grieving*.

6. Jan Richardson, *The Cure for Sorrow: A Book of Blessings for Times of Grief* (Orlando: Wanton Gospeller Press, 2020).

About the Authors

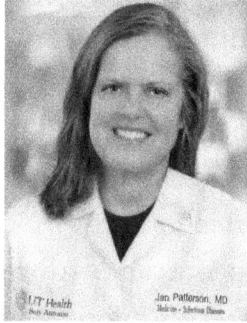

Jan E. Patterson, MD, MS, is an integrative medicine and infectious diseases physician who has been in academic medical practice for more than thirty years. She graduated from McGovern Medical School in Houston, did her residency in internal medicine at Vanderbilt University Medical Center in Nashville, and her fellowship in infectious diseases at Yale University School of Medicine in New Haven, Connecticut. After several years on the faculty at Yale, she and her husband, also an infectious diseases physician, returned to Texas and have been on the faculty at the Long School of Medicine, UT Health San Antonio for more than twenty-five years. She is currently professor of medicine/infectious diseases and associate dean for quality and lifelong learning there. She is the medical director of integrative medicine at the affiliated health system, University Health.

Dr. Patterson completed a master's in Health Care Management at Harvard School of Public Health and has held medical leadership positions at the local and regional level, as well as at the national level in her professional societies. Her continued interest in additional ways to help patients led her to complete a fellowship in integrative medicine at the Andrew Weil Center for Integrative Medicine at University of Arizona.

She has continued to provide care for patients throughout her career, as well as work in health-care epidemiology and infection prevention, clinical research, health-care improvement and education of health-care professionals, fellows, residents, and medical students. She is the author of more than 150 scientific publications. She has been an invited speaker in local, regional, national, and international venues, and has received honors and awards for her work and service throughout her career.

Dr. Patterson is a native of Fort Worth, Texas, and has been married to the inimitable Dr. Thomas Patterson for thirty-six years. She is the mother of two sons and two dogs and enjoys gardening and being outdoors in her spare time.

Website: https://www.drjanpatterson.com
Twitter: @drjanpatterson

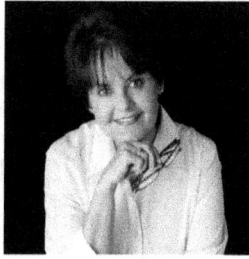

Phyllis Clark Nichols's writing and her character-driven southern fiction explore profound human questions using the imagined residents of small-town communities you just know you've visited before. With a strong faith and a love for nature, art, music, and ordinary people, she tells redemptive tales of loss and recovery, estrangement and connection, longing and fulfillment...often through surprisingly serendipitous events. She is the author of eleven books, including The Rockwater Suite series and The Family Portrait series.

Phyllis's nonfiction book *Sacred Sense from Taking a Second Look* was a Selah Award Winner for Audiobooks. *Searching for the Song*, the fifth book in her Rockwater Suite, was a finalist in the Inspirational Fiction category in the International Book Awards Competition.

Phyllis grew up in the deep shade of magnolia trees in South Georgia. In addition to her life as a writer, she is a seminary graduate, pianist, soprano soloist, and cofounder of a national cable network with health-and disability-related programming. She performs musical monologues that express her faith, joy, and thoughts about life—all with the homespun humor and gentility of a true southern woman. Regardless of her role, Phyllis brings creativity and compelling storytelling.

Phyllis currently serves on two nonprofit boards. She loves cooking, travel, music, the arts, and the great outdoors. She lives in the Texas Hill Country with her portrait-artist, theologian husband, Dr. Bill Nichols.

Website: PhyllisClarkNichols.com
Facebook: facebook.com/Phyllis Clark Nichols
Twitter: @PhyllisCNichols

www.ingramcontent.com/pod-product-compliance
Lightning Source LLC
Chambersburg PA
CBHW050108280326
41933CB00010B/1021